MW00908792

Also by

Lewis G. Maharam, M.D., FACSM

———————

Maharam's Curve: The Exercise High—
How to Get It, How to Keep It

A
HEALTHY BACK

A Sports Medicine Doctor's
Back-Care Program
for Every *BODY*

• • • • • • •

Lewis G. Maharam,
M.D., FACSM

An Owl Book
Henry Holt and Company   •   New York

Henry Holt and Company, Inc.
Publishers since 1866
115 West 18th Street
New York, New York 10011

Henry Holt® is a registered trademark
of Henry Holt and Company, Inc.

Copyright © 1996 by Lewis G. Maharam, M.D., FACSM
All rights reserved.
Published in Canada by Fitzhenry & Whiteside Ltd.,
195 Allstate Parkway, Markham, Ontario L3R 4T8.

Library of Congress Cataloging-in-Publication Data
Maharam, Lewis G.
[Backs in motion]
A healthy back: a sports medicine doctor's back-care
for everyBody / Lewis G. Maharam.—1st Owl Books ed.
p.   cm.
Previously published as: Backs in motion. 1996.
"An Owl Book."
Includes index.
ISBN 0-8050-3541-9
1. Backache—Exercise therapy.   2. Back—Care and hygiene.
3. Backache—Prevention.   4. Athletes—Health and hygiene.
I. Title.
RD771.B217M34   1996   97-43020
617.5'64—dc21   CIP

Henry Holt books are available for special promotions and
premiums. For details contact: Director, Special Markets.

First published in hardcover as *Backs in Motion*
in 1996 by Henry Holt and Company, Inc.

First Owl Books Edition 1998

Designed by Victoria Hartman

Printed in the United States of America
All first editions are printed on acid-free paper.∞

1   3   5   7   9   10   8   6   4   2

To Welabucs . . .

Who Knew . . .

Acknowledgments

Balance. Between treating patients, covering sporting events, giving lectures, as well as organizing and attending sports medicine conferences, it was a challenge to schedule time to thought-pack and research this book. I am grateful to many special people for their belief and understanding in my work.

Thanks to my ace agent Joan Raines and her team of Theron and Keith at Raines and Raines who cheered me along.

Sincere thanks to my editor Cynthia Vartan at Henry Holt and Company, Inc., for her enthusiasm and guidance; Claudia Lory Koziol, P.T., the physical therapist's physical therapist; Allan M. Levy, M.D., for his friendship and vision; and John A. Delves III, editor of *Masters Sports* newsletter, my one-man thesaurus.

The writing of this book was made more pleasurable by the encouragement of colleagues and sports medicine professionals. Many thanks to: Bob Adams, D.O.; Phillip A. Bauman, M.D.; Louis U. Bigliani, M.D.; David A. Birnbaum, M.D.; C. Harmon Brown, M.D.; Robert C. Cantu, M.D.; Micheline Cerra, P.T.; Jerry L. Cochran, M.D.; Harold M. Dick, M.D.; Kenneth Ermann, D.C.; Hugh H. Gardy, D.D.S.; Ronald P. Grelsamer, M.D.; Stuart J. Hershon, M.D.; Barry D. Jordan, M.D.; Kevin Kennedy, P.T., A.T.,C.; Joseph Kolb, A.T.,C.; David S. Levesque, D.P.M.; Adrian Lorde, B.Sc., M.B.B.S., M.Sc.(UWI); Ellen L. Marmer, M.D.; Stephen J. McIlveen, M.D.; John E. McNerney, D.P.M.; Lyle J. Micheli, M.D.; Michael Minardo, D.C.; Sandy Minardo; Gabe Mirkin, M.D.; Kevin Moody, A.T.,C.; Michael G. Neuwirth, M.D.; Stephen M. Perle, D.C.; Mark I. Pitman, M.D.; Kalmon Post, M.D.; Stephen G. Rice, M.D., Ph.D., M.P.H.; Andres Rodriguez, M.D.; Yolanda Rodriguez; Melvin P. Rosenwasser, M.D.; Jack Russell, D.O.; Joseph S. Sanfilippo, M.D.; Abby Corsun Sims, P.T.; Heidi Skolnick, M.S.; Susan L. Snouse, A.T.,C.; and Jim Whitehead.

I am also grateful to my treasured friends: Nicholas Barbaro; Ian Brooks; Joe Caruso; Stella Cashman; Hon. Stephen G. Crane; Frederick N. Gaffney, Esq.; Phillip Greenwald; Roz Katz; Ron Lombardi; Caryn Mack; Richard Mack, D.O.; Shymal Majumdar, Ph.D.; Rick Pascarella; G. Earl Peace, Ph.D.; Sue Polansky; Nancy Preiser; Pat and Helio Rico; Rudy Riska; John Roselli; Wade Silverman, Ph.D.; Tracy Sundlun; Billy Taylor; and Bruce Weddell, Esq.

Extra thanks to: Andrea and Tom Plate as well as my precious goddaughter Ashley Plate; my caring in-laws Norma and Leonard Michelson; and Bobby, Ann, Maggie, and Joel Michelson. And of course, huge thanks to my loving wife Marcia, my lovely grandmother Bebe, my mother Jane from whom all goodness comes, and my best friend/sister Patsy, and kisses and hugs to my Eddy boy.

Contents

Introduction

Hippocrates used electric eels to relieve back muscle spasms. We don't do that anymore. Modern medicine has provided us with far more sophisticated—not to mention less slimy—ways of treating bad backs, ways that would have amazed Hippocrates. What would have amazed him even more, however, is that for all our sophistication, eight out of ten Americans still struggle with back pain. Most of our modern solutions aren't working.

But that's changing. We're finally beginning to understand the importance of one simple fact, a fact that opens up new avenues of prevention and treatment: the spine has a life of its own.

Your back is dynamic—it *moves*.

Pretty obvious when you think about it. After all, every time you breathe, it heaves obligingly up and down, inward and outward. Put on your shoes and it rounds for-

1

ward. Hug a child and it obediently expands to both sides. When you walk, talk, even when you sleep, it's moving.

But that's not how we've traditionally been taught to see this important—and in far too many cases, temperamental—part of our body. Until now, almost everybody thought of the spine as a static rod, a long, steely tower of interlocking bone. Yet look around you. The man lugging his gym bag down the street is listing to the left like a sailboat, leaning to his tote-carrying side. The "sedentary" receptionist in the office? Her spine will twist as she reaches across the desk to answer the phone. Then, because like most of us, she doesn't sit stick-straight, it will round back into a slight curve as she settles into her chair.

Standing, sitting, making your bed, doing the laundry, your back moves—left, right, forward, backward. And that's just during your everyday motions. Imagine what it does when you swing a golf club, ride a bike, pitch a softball, or serve a tennis ball.

So it's a highly supple stack of bones that separates your head from your bottom, a fact that has everything to do with how I propose to keep it healthy and strong. What we now understand about the spine's flowing dynamics has created nothing less than a revolution in preventing and treating back pain. And what I want to teach you about your back is going to revolutionize your own personal approach to keeping fit and staying active. If you've been told that back pain is something you'll "just have to live with," don't believe it. You can prevent back pain, and you can alleviate it if you're already troubled. With the Backs in Motion program in this book, I guarantee you will.

The breakthrough came originally from sports medicine, a relatively new specialty for active people that has taken huge strides over the last ten years toward injury prevention and treatment. As a doctor, that's precisely what attracted me to it. It's helped us better understand torn ligaments and "blown-out" knees. And it's helped us better understand backs, too, by looking not just at their structure but at their biomechanics, not just how they're *built*, but what they *do*. At last we no longer think of the back as frozen in place.

It took a team physician for a professional football club to sound the wake-up call. Early in my career, I was an associate of Dr. Allan Levy, a pioneering sports medicine physician and team doctor for the New York Giants. Like so many established professionals, Dr. Levy had his hands full with the usual carnage of his specialty—broken bones, pulled muscles, shredded tendons, dislocated shoulders. The back was too temperamental, and the most effective treatments still too theoretical, for him to do the thorough job he wanted without investing more research time than he had to spare. But as a freshman M.D., I sure had the time. I also had the curiosity. So when "Doc" Levy asked me to handle all of the back patients, he didn't have to ask twice.

I devoured everything in sight about the back, and sat in on conference after conference on back care. Early on I came to believe that the study of biomechanics—the body in motion—would be the key to providing a complete back-care program, and that sports medicine could find that key. What I also learned is that while there are thousands of reasons for back pain, if you look hard enough, you'll find the one that's causing it. It's an obsession I like to call being "compulsively diagnostic." Good sports medicine is as compulsive as they come.

If you've ever been diagnosed as having "low back pain," you know how athletes used to feel when they hurt themselves. Before sports medicine, physicians used to tell peple with knee injuries that they had "internal derangement of the knee"—a handy catchall that could translate into the equally fuzzy "uh-oh, you have a bad knee." They would then warn against any cycling, or tennis, or running for a while, and suggest a general set of exercises in the hope that things would get better. With their limited diagnostic tools, they could hardly have done otherwise.

We can do better now, for knees, for ankles, for shoulders—and for backs. Now, through the use of MRIs, CT myelograms, and high-tech arthrograms, we can diagnose tiny individual ligament tears and tell patients exactly what's wrong, and design an exacting treatment plan based on that diagnosis. We don't give you all-purpose exercises or other therapies anymore, we give you specific ones. We give you *yours*.

Tony, a tax accountant who came to see me with back pain he couldn't shake, is a classic example. His family physician had sternly warned him that his back pain was a result of his running twenty miles a week. "Stop running and your back pain will go away," the doctor said. Probably true, but Tony didn't like that answer. Running made him so happy!

So Tony came to see me. He had heard that, as Medical Director for the Metropolitan Athletics Congress, the New York association for U.S. Track & Field, I was particularly interested in runners, so I was his last hope. "Doc," he shook his head sadly, "I don't want to stop running, but it hurts. Every day in the office I feel stiff. I sit with a pillow behind my back, but that doesn't help. I pop Motrin and Advil. It stays the same. So now I'm here."

Sports medicine has taught us over and over that what actually hurts may be far away from what's causing the pain, so we probe around. After doing an examination, I could comfortably give Tony the answer he had hoped for. Running was not his back problem. His legs were his back problem. "You have a leg-length discrepancy that's making your back muscles work overtime," I told him. "And yes, there is something you can do about it." When both legs are not identical in length, the runner's pelvis has to wobble left and right to compensate, straining muscles that can ultimately go into spasm. Tony's had done just that. My Backs in Motion recommendation was a series of exercises that would stretch and strengthen those specific muscles to eliminate the spasming, followed by orthotics or shoe inserts that would even his legs up and keep the problem from coming back. That's all Tony had to hear. Last time I saw him, he and his orthotics were training for the New York City Marathon.

In one sense his family doctor was right: running twenty miles a week was part of Tony's problem, not because it's a lot for a runner but because his back wasn't prepared to deal with his anatomical flaw. And looking beyond the "low back pain" all-purpose expediency let us lick the trouble.

Of course if your back isn't prepared for it, you don't even have to have a mechanical flaw to suffer the strain of athletic activity, or even the strain of an everyday movement like running for a bus, raking leaves, or making beds. When right-handed actor John Goodman was making the movie *The Babe,* he trained hard for the role. But as soon as he got up to bat, he hurt his back anyway. Trying to accurately portray Babe Ruth, it turns out, he had switched from batting righty to batting lefty. He suddenly needed flexibility and strength on the left side, but he didn't have it because all of his training had instinctively focused on the right.

But a word of warning: even though we know far more today about how our bodies really move, and how to keep them strong enough for those motions, that doesn't mean all back problems will yield to mechanical or muscular changes. Most people can mend with the help of an active program, but obviously not everyone can. If exercise alone were the answer, world-class competitors like Olympic marathoners Pete Pfitzinger and Anne Audain would never have been sidelined with bad backs. Unfortunately there will always be people who cannot benefit from an exercise program or physical therapy. I view surgery as a last resort— the failure of all other treatments to work—but some people do require it to get better. If your back problem is that severe and you have chronic pain, then this isn't the program for you. However, if you're like the majority of the patients I see—active, and wanting to stay that way—you'll do well with the Backs in Motion program.

You can even keep your back, in a sense, younger. As we age, certain unavoidable physical changes occur in our spines. The disks that separate and cushion our vertebrae degenerate, shrinking in size, flattening out and losing their shock absorbing capacity, increasing the likelihood that the bones will press on or rub a nerve. *Ouch!* Some of us also develop arthritis in the joints, limiting our backs' range of motion. While nothing can stop those changes, this program can help you remain strong and flexible, giving you the best chance of minimizing their effect. Whether your back troubles come from an injury or simply from the aging process, there is most likely a solution for what ails you, and it's now right at your fingertips.

Considering the statistics—two-thirds of Americans have been incapacitated by back pain at least once—it's easy to see how what I call the great back myth got started. An equal-opportunity injury calls for an equal-opportunity solution, so the convenient myth says that everybody can be helped by the same classic half dozen exercises that back books and doctors all recommend. They are effective exercises, to be sure, but they only lay the foundation.

The reason is that what ails my back is not necessarily what ails yours. When patients come to see me, the first thing I ask them is what sport or activity they take part in most frequently. Do they walk? Kneel in the garden, weeding? Ride a bike? Play tennis? Or do they mostly just walk up and down the stairs at home or the office? I'm not as curious about how much they move as I am about *how* they move. Are they frequently twisting their torso to swing a golf club? Are their hamstrings being yanked forward on their daily five-mile run? Or are their lower back muscles being tugged on via a leash several times a day by Sally, the lumbering Labrador retriever who never learned the meaning of "heel!"? These are important distinctions because they determine which parts of the body need to be prepped in order to take strain off the back.

Today we know that exercise plays a crucial role in preventing and relieving back pain. In fact, just about every physician, physical therapist, and back book author prescribes exercises to people with back problems. The only trouble is—in much the same way that "internal derangement of the knee" was once used as an all-purpose stick-on label—they've been prescribing those same six stretching and strengthening exercises to everyone. No matter that your cousin plays basketball three nights a week and your husband watches TV. No matter that Aunt Ruth suffers from a herniated disk and Uncle Al from spinal stenosis. They all get the same prescription. Good-bye and good luck.

My exercise program is different. While I'm not going to throw the familiar six exercises out the window, I want to give you a new perspective on them. They are the *foundation* of a healthy back program, not its substance. You need to build on them. So along with those classic six— plus two that also help lay the groundwork—I'm going to give you exercises that will prepare your back for the specific demands you make on it. Do you run? Do you walk to work each day? Are you a cyclist? There's a conditioning program that suits your particular needs.

Why doesn't one exercise program fit all? Think for a moment about how your body moves when you swing a golf club as opposed to how it moves when you shoot a basket or bend down to pick up a box. Every sport and even every domestic activity, from walking the dog to carrying a child, stresses the back in a particular and unique way. While being generally fit can help you handle those stresses, you can weather them much better if the muscles that surround and support the spine have been conditioned to take the exact moves you'll be making.

It's not much different from practicing a sport. A squash player must do different conditioning exercises to prepare his back than a swimmer, who must do different things than a runner, who must do different things than a weight lifter. The Backs in Motion program is so named not only because it prescribes activity as a remedy for back pain, but because it's designed to anticipate motion and prevent pain by preparing the muscles. Many of the exercises you'll find in this book mimic the movements demanded by activity, so that you're not just stretching and strengthening, you're also readying the muscles to move in the direction you'll need them to go. By the time the golfer tees off or the cyclist hunkers down and pedals, the muscles for those actions will have been primed to protect, rather than stress, the back.

Even if your toughest workout is hauling the month's recyclables up from the basement, you still need to prep for the movements you make most frequently. Often you can do that by using some of the same exercises athletes use: The muscles used to spike a volleyball over the net are the same ones that help you pick a can of vegetables off the top cupboard shelf. Pushing a vacuum is not very different from pulling an oar. You can prepare for these everyday activities. You can even prepare for sex, which in my book is just like any other sport—including positions that are good for making the play and ones that are risky.

As long as your back-priming routine is as specific as possible, you're in business.

The program on the following pages is designed to address your specific needs. It's individualized. And it's detailed. Golfer, runner, ballroom-dancing grandma, tennis player, or woodcarver, you'll find exactly what will help you mend a bad back or keep a good one healthy.

You'll also find help with the obvious question: what's actually *wrong* with your back, anyway? As with any complex piece of machinery that has moveable parts, you've got to know what's "broke" before you can properly fix it; the next two chapters are devoted to helping you do that. I'm not going to diagnose you or encourage you to diagnose yourself. No book should ever substitute for a doctor's care, and this one isn't meant to. What I can do, however, is give you the information you need to be an informed consumer. After reading this book, you'll walk into your doctor's office, ask the right questions, and walk out with an exact diagnosis—or, if not, you'll know it's time to find somebody who's willing to give you one.

That's all my patient Janet, a fifty-three-year-old college professor, needed to get back in the weight room. Someone had to find out how, and why, her exercise program and her back disagreed. She had the stamina of a woman half her age, thanks to regular workouts on her gym's Cybex machines and some calisthenics classes. But oh, that backache! Was she overdoing it at her age, she worried?

No, I told her, the problem actually started when she was a kid—probably at conception. She had a condition called spinal stenosis, which means the canal the spinal cord travels through is too small, subjecting the nerves there to irritating friction during some motions, such as extreme extensions and flexions of the trunk. All we had to do was switch her from sit-ups to crunches, which use a smaller range of motion, and limit her extensions on the weight machines. I was in her gym one day and there she was, smiling up at me from the seated rowing machine, sweating buckets and loving it.

But to help you, I need your help. Football coach Bill Parcells used to say that he didn't win ball games by himself. What he did was put the players in the best position to make the play; they had to go out and do it. In this book, I'm going to give you all the information you need to put together your own game plan. For you to be pain-free, you'll have to make the play yourself.

But at least you won't have to sit in a chair to make it, no matter how many times you've heard the old wive's tale that active people have more back problems than inactive people do. No, they don't. Though sedentary people like to believe that never sweating somehow protects them, in fact it's just the opposite. Their muscles are unprepared for their motions of everyday life, and something as simple as hoisting their carry-on luggage into an airplane's over-head compartment may be all it takes to produce an injury. For the most part, athletes as well as people who move a great deal during the day are stronger and more flexible than people who don't. If they do weight-bearing exercise, they also have a decreased risk of osteoporosis, a bone-thinning disease that can bring about back pain.

Exercise increases blood circulation, insuring that the disks and nerves in your back are well nourished with oxy-gen and essential nutrients. And since excess pounds can put stress on your spine, exercise's role in weight mainte-nance is another plus. So while an avid cyclist may subject her back to more wear and tear than someone whose main sport is channel surfing, her body is also better equipped to handle it.

The conditioning exercises ahead will help prevent back pain from occurring and alleviate pain you already have. They'll do something else, too: help you approach activity intelligently. Some athletes I've seen in my office have shrugged off back problems, contending that they're the price one has to pay for being active. Pain or no pain, these martyrs continue training at the same breakneck pace. Then there are the people who work out until it hurts, at which point they give up everything until the pain goes away—or for good, because they're too afraid of what may happen in the future. What you'll learn here is that you don't have to be a martyr or a quitter: there *is* a happy medium.

The reason I enjoy sports medicine so much is that I get to work with people who are dedicated to getting better fast. They pitch in willingly in their own treatment. If you have read this far, I know that you too are willing to do what it takes to get back in action. I'm going to tell you exactly what that is, but first, an anatomy lesson to give you the basic knowledge you need before we set the ball in play. Let's begin . . .

PART I

A
Back
Owner's
Manual

... *1* ...

Your Back Comes
with Moveable Parts:
A New Anatomy Lesson

This is the first step in your journey to a strong, healthy, pain-free back. Like all important journeys, it's going to take us through unfamiliar territory, and like a tourist in a foreign country, you're going to need a basic, working vocabulary. Nothing fancy, mind you, just the anatomical equivalent of "Drive me back to my hotel by the shortest route, please," or "Where is the nearest public bathroom?" or "Waiter, may I have the check?" Basic tools for getting along. So welcome to the Maharam School of Anatomical Language, Department of Backs. I'll be your professor for the next few pages. Some of what we have to cover may seem a little musty, but when we're done, you'll speak "back" fluently enough to get the most out of your trip.

But before we start, reach for the eraser and rub out the old anatomy poster image of your back that you may have in your mind: a bunch of knobby little bones stacked one on top of the other, plunging like a rod from your neck to your rear, stiff and static.

Looks can be deceiving. We need a new model to better understand what the back allows us to do and what can happen to it. And the image you need to have in mind to use my program successfully is that of a straw in the middle of a cup. The straw represents your spine—its vertebrae, disks, and nerves. The cup is your trunk, with its muscles, tendons, and ligaments. The stronger the cup, the better protected the straw. The stronger your trunk, the safer your spine. There, we're already through with lesson one. Now that wasn't so hard, was it?

However, lesson two is more involved, because it shows how well designed the straw is for the hundreds of little ways it moves, thereby keeping us from looking like welded robots as we move this way and that through the day. While the spine pictured on that old anatomy poster may look rigid, some of those knobs are really joints that, with a gliding motion, allow the spine to shift in small but varied ways. Others are levers attached to muscles that make those movements possible in the first place. Without the joints and levers shifting around, you couldn't swing a bat, throw a football, make a bed.

So the back and its muscles are always in motion. But what happens when the muscles and joints are not adequately strong or flexible? For instance, if a golfer has paid no particular attention to his trunk muscles, the ones that bring the club back and down to fire through the swing, what happens? And let's think about what happens to a runner's back if the hamstring muscles that flex his leg with every stride do not have enough give. Since the muscles ultimately connect to the spine and help accomplish day-to-day movements, tight ones can yank the spine instead and trigger pain.

When you become well versed in biomechanics—the movements a given sport requires of your body parts—you also better understand what causes or exacerbates your back pain. But first you need to know the parts themselves.

With the availability of general information today, it is hard not to have heard of disks, vertebrae, ligaments, and the sciatic nerve. But by the time we're done, you'll know how each functions in both the day-to-day and sports-specific moves you make. You'll understand not just your back's anatomy, but its biomechanics. And what it needs to do the job well.

But the real question is, how will all of this help you get rid of back pain or prevent you from getting it in the first place? As a sports medicine physician, I can say we need to take our lessons from athletes, the men and women who are probably the best medical consumers around. Driven by the determination to get back in action after something sidelines them, athletes often go to great lengths to learn about their bodies. When a doctor identifies what's wrong, athletes not only understand it, they also understand exactly why the specific treatment was prescribed and what it is designed to do. And if one doctor can't tell them precisely what's wrong, they look for another who can. As anatomy "experts," they understand the importance of getting a very specific diagnosis.

Even if you are not an athlete, learning how your back works will give you the same kind of edge that professional athletes have been taking advantage of for years. Not only will your knowledge help you take care of your back, but along the way it will also give you more insight into the quality of medical care you're getting.

Later in this book I'm going to give you an exercise program that will require diligence and perseverance. And I'm betting you'll stick to it. Because after reading this chapter and the one that follows, you're going to know not only why you're doing the exercises I prescribe but why it's important to make them a part of your daily life, whether you are an athlete, a mom, a musician, or a student. Finally and most essentially, you'll be a partner in your own health care.

So let's start at the top, or in this case, the center.

Your Elegant "S"

There's no other bony structure in the body with the finesse of your spine. It's an elaborate tower constructed primarily of vertebrae, the disks between them, the spinal cord running through the vertebrae, nerves, blood vessels, and the ligaments that hold everything together. To get an idea of how elegantly these parts are arranged, stand sideways in front of a mirror. Notice how your back is shaped like an elongated "S"? Those natural, springlike curves distribute the weight of your head and torso and enable your spine to absorb shock better. Jump off a stool with your legs locked, and you'll feel the jolt of hitting the floor right up to the fillings in your teeth. Do it again with knees bent, and your body easily and gracefully absorbs the force. Same thing with the spine. If it were arrow-straight, the lower vertebrae would have to bear the cumulative weight and impact of everything piled on top of them. A curving structure spreads the load out more evenly (see figure 1.1).

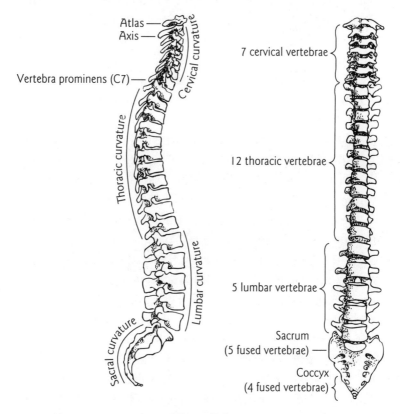

Figure 1.1

If only we didn't have gravity getting in the way, the "S" would be more graceful yet. To see a perfectly curved back, on this planet at least, someone would have to hold you by the ears and dangle you in a deep-water pool. Only as you floated straight up and down, motionless and without the weight of gravity, would your spine finally hang with its natural curves perfectly aligned (figure 1.1): the slight forward rounding of the upper back (*kyphosis*), the backward pitch of the lower spine (*lordosis*), even the slight tilt it adopts when you lean sideways (*scoliosis*).

But of course we don't live in pools, and we don't stand still much either, so our spine's curves are always a little "off." Leaning forward exaggerates the upper back curve (kyphosis); bending backward increases the lower back curve (lordosis); and stretching way out to the side forms an exaggerated sideways curve (scoliosis). Though the shapes are normal and the motions are all in a day's work for most spines, the curves should be neither extreme nor persistent. When they reach that degree, they're considered abnormal.

Arcane? Even I thought the terms were a little obscure for my patients until one day I began slowly explaining them to a great-grandmother in her mid-eighties who was seeing me for chronic back pain. "Oh, I know all about that already" she cut me off, eyes twinkling. "When I was at Wellesley, none of my friends could remember the three names for spinal curvatures. Our anatomy exam was the next day, and we were desperate for a good grade, so we hit on the idea of turning them into a football cheer." And with that, the fire came into her eyes—she was up on her feet and back in her dorm room in Massachusetts sixty-some years ago instead of in my office. "Ky-*pho*-sis! [forward she went], lor-*do*-sis! [torso thrown back], sco-li-*o*-sis! [skewed to the side], *flat feet!!*" she chanted with go-get-'em-guys rhythm and perfectly matching spinal tilts, toes splayed out for the finale. (See figure 1.2.) I still don't know how "flat feet" got in there, but she wasn't put off by doctorspeak and she knew her anatomy. So can you.

Know, too, that these slight exaggerations aren't unhealthy; they're part of the body's natural range of motion. Nonetheless, each time the spine deviates from its normal "S" shape, it's not in the best position to distribute the body's weight with its natural kyphosis and lordosis. If, for instance, you're always sitting with your spine curved to the side, or standing with your upper back hunched, the unequal distribution of weight over time can take its toll. And anything that increases the load, like regularly carrying

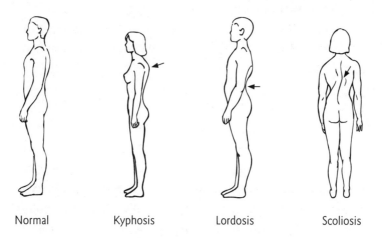

Normal   Kyphosis   Lordosis   Scoliosis

Figure 1.2

your three-year-old on one hip, will weigh even more heavily on your vertebrae and disks. Likewise, physical activity can add to the stress, since movement, even seemingly easy movement, such as walking, also loads the spine. But it does so naturally, because, craving stability, your body constantly tries to maintain a line of gravity, an imaginary straight path running right down its center. When movement or anything else disrupts that balance, muscles work to restore it. Not necessarily a hard job, but one they must be ready to do over and over. And although most people's lordotic, kyphotic, and scoliotic curves are exaggerated only for short periods of time, for some backs the abnormal degree is permanent. In these abnormal instances where a congenital (and often hereditary) structure is present, the "S" curves are always out of optimum alignment and eventually cause pain—that is, unless strategic muscles are targeted for extra strengthening to help the body cope with increased balancing responsibilities.

So that's the spine, absorbing shocks and fighting gravity every step of the way. But how does the spine really do that?

Vertebrae: The Primary
Pieces of the Puzzle

If you compare the vertebrae to, say, the bones in your arm or leg, the vertebrae seem pretty dinky. Don't be fooled. Each of these bone-and-cartilage structures is extremely complex and, together with the ones above and below, creates a pillar of both stability and movement: the spine. Small in size, but big in versatility and strength.

Adults have thirty-three vertebrae (twenty-four of which move), named for the part of the spine where they're found (see figure 1.1). Seven make up the cervical (neck) region of the spine, twelve are thoracic (upper back), and five are lumbar (lower back). Five more are fused together to form what's called the sacrum in the pelvic region and the last four, also fused together, form your coccyx, or tailbone.

Handily, each vertebra has a name or, you might say, a coordinate. C1 refers to the first cervical vertebra, obviously in the neck; L5 is the fifth lumbar vertebra; and so on. Logically, the disks between the vertebrae are referred to by the name of the "sandwich" they're in; L4-5 is between the fourth and fifth lumbar vertebrae, for example.

It's no surprise that in a column that does as much as the spine, no two vertebrae are identical. Depending on where they're located, they perform different jobs. Cervical vertebrae, for instance, are smaller and more delicate than the ones lower down because, while they support your head—as well as allow it to rotate—they don't support much else. The thoracic vertebrae immediately below are bigger. Once upon a time it was thought that since they're attached to and somewhat restricted by the ribs, they don't have much to do with body movement. Now we know better, thanks to more precise functional studies of the body. Try twisting around to look behind you, or leaning one elbow on the table, your head over to one side. Your upper back moves, and it moves plenty. Thank your thoracic vertebrae, and the many muscles of your upper back that attach to them, for this mobility.

And finally, we have what I call the high-risk, high-reward vertebrae: the lumbars. These guys *really* move. Nature has made them the most massive of all to bear the brunt of the torso's weight, when you dive to the side to return a tennis serve or rotate your torso in the freestyle swimming stroke. When you use your boardinghouse reach to grab the potatoes or arch dreamily backward to savor the sky on a starry night, the lumbars are working for you. All of this movement, though, plus the weight that's piled on the lumbar vertebrae, make them the vertebrae most at risk. To a lot of people, "back pain" begins and ends with lumbar pain.

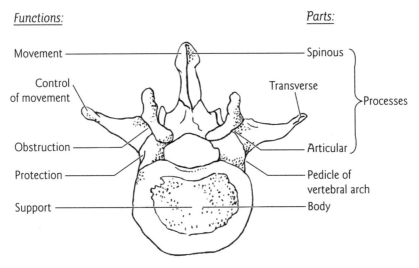

Figure 1.3

Variable though they all are, most vertebrae have two sections that look as though they've been fused together (see figure 1.3). The front part, which faces the front of your body, is an oval slice of bone called the vertebral body. Broad and solid, it bears most of the weight of your upper body: 90 percent of it when you're sitting down, maybe 10 percent less when you're standing.

But the back half is not to be outdone. Made of bone and cartilage, this half looks like an arch with three prongs protruding from the rear. Without the back half, your spinal cord would be destroyed. For chief among the functions of this piece of bone is to shelter the body's lifeline.

At the point where the back half and front half of the vertebra meet, they form a triangular opening to house the spinal cord, nerves, and blood vessels. Since the vertebrae are stacked one on top of the other, the consecutive openings create a protective vertical canal for these fragile structures, a safe passageway running from the brain all the way down to the second lumbar vertebra.

Along the way, other openings allow nerves to exit to the side, nerves that control different parts of the leg. At the bottom of the spine, the nerves that are left coalesce into the famous sciatic nerve, which travels down the leg.

This intricate weave of nerves and bone is often the source of back pain. If, for instance, the spinal canal narrows, or one of the side openings closes in slightly, bone can rub against nerve. A chafed nerve becomes an inflamed nerve, which in turn becomes a painful nerve. And the process is so specific that a doctor can often tell which nerve is being affected just by knowing where your pain is.

Now, just behind that protective spinal cord column are the three prongs technically called processes. Their main job is to attach the spinal column to muscles and ligaments, meaning they not only work to help support the spine, they are the handles the muscles tug on when they want to move the spine. By the way, you feel the middle, or spinous, process protruding down the center of your back as a bony knob just below the skin.

Obviously the vertebrae can't just sit there perched on top of each other doing all of this important work. Something has to connect them, and something does. Ligaments—fibrous, slightly elastic bands—run down their sides, essentially stringing them together and keeping them from going too far when you bend one way or another.

Your Most Moveable Parts: The Tri-Joint Complex

But ligaments alone don't hold the vertebrae together either. Three joints do a lot of the work: a disk sandwiched between the vertebral bodies that functions enough like a joint to be considered one, and two so-called facet joints that connect the back (pronged) parts of the vertebrae together (see figure 1.4)—one to the vertebra below, the other to the one above. The facet joint moves only slightly, but the cumulative effect of each one doing that adds up to a huge range of motion for you, allowing a pitcher to rotate

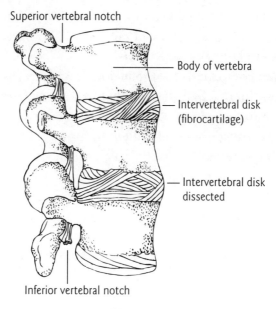

Superior vertebral notch

Body of vertebra

Intervertebral disk (fibrocartilage)

Intervertebral disk dissected

Inferior vertebral notch

Figure 1.4

as he unleashes a fast ball or a rower to bend forward to pull the oar through the water. Even when you stoop to turn the water on in the bathtub, the three-joint complex is at work. And although we've understood the basic mechanics for years, only recently have we begun to appreciate the starring role the three-joint complex plays in keeping the back healthy. Here's why.

The Disks

The disks are your body's shock absorbers, roundish pads that are sandwiched between two vertebrae to prevent bone from hitting bone. They also function like joints, as we said, because they keep the vertebrae cushioned and able to bend forward as you cut loose a bowling ball or cock backward in a tennis serve.

I often compare disks to jelly doughnuts, because that's just what they're like (see figure 1.5) with their relatively hard exteriors and soft insides. The doughnut's "crust" is a layered cartilaginous shell called the annulus fibrosus, the "jelly" a gelatinlike substance called the nucleus pulposus. It's that soft, gelatinous, plumped-up nucleus that gives the disk its shock-absorbing power and keeps the vertebrae raised off each other and aligned so that weight is properly distributed among them.

The secret ingredient that lets a disk do so much? Water. Molecules inside the nucleus, called proteoglycans, are the largest molecules in the human body and also the thirstiest. These molecules are able to increase their weight 250 times simply by drinking up water from the body. When we are children, that is exactly what the disk molecules do. In fact, when we are in our thirties, the disks are still composed of about 90 percent water. As we grow older, the percent gradually declines, and though that's not good news for most of us, it doesn't necessarily have to

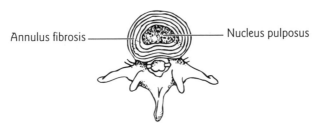

Annulus fibrosis ———— Nucleus pulposus

Figure 1.5

be bad news either. (We'll talk about disk difficulties in the next chapter.)

The Facet Joints

When you think about a joint, the hingelike elbow or knee, or possibly the ball-and-socket design of the hip, come to mind. Most people don't realize that any cartilage-lined surface moving against another surface and attached to a muscle is a "joint" in medical parlance. There's a lesser-known kind of joint you may never have heard of: the gliding joint. Nothing complicated about it, the gliding joint works just like it sounds—one part glides over the other. Put your two index fingers together skin to skin and gently rub the foreparts up and down against each other. You've just demonstrated a gliding joint.

The facets are gliding joints (see figure 1.6). They aren't designed for the kind of big, dramatic motions that hinge

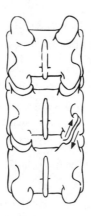

Figure 1.6

or ball-and-socket joints are capable of, but the movements they do perform let you bend and rotate. The facet joints fundamentally control how far and in which direction you can move.

But that's not all. Clever little load bearers that they are, as the facet joints move, they also take some of the pressure off the disks, helping to keep the disks healthy. At the same time the facet joints play the spinal disciplinarian, working to keep everything in the column aligned. And you don't want them to fail at this, for if any of the facet joints get out of line, the vertebrae above and below are likely to follow.

Also Starring: The Back Muscles

Without muscles, there is no motion anywhere—including the back. Muscles, as you know, connect bones across joints. When they contract, voilà! Motion. Though they're usually discussed only peripherally in descriptions of how the back works, in point of fact, your back can't work without them.

As I say to patients, if something has to go wrong, let it be the muscles. When one of the back's primary structures fails—vertebrae, disks, facet joints—recovery can be time consuming and complicated. But most back problems are muscle problems—pulls, strains, sprains—and dealing with those is far less daunting.

Don't worry, we won't labor through a complete list of back muscles because there are scads of them: long ones,

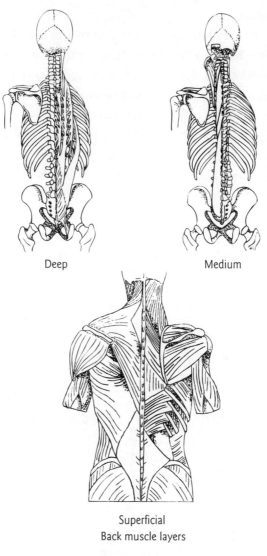

Deep   Medium

Superficial
Back muscle layers

Figure 1.7

short ones, medium ones. Plus layers! Three of those: deep, medium, and superficial. Just realize that the chance that something, sometime, will put a strain on one of those muscles is not small, even though people persist in blaming their back pain on something much more complicated, scaring themselves half to death in the process.

Most muscle trouble is easy to prevent. Muscles that are stretched and flexible have give. They allow you to move with ease and comfort. And they act in concert with the disks and the elongated "S" to absorb shock (see figure 1.8).

But suppleness can't do it all. Having strong back muscles is as important as having stretched ones, since part of the back muscles' job is to support the weight of the trunk loaded on the spine. Remember the cup and straw analogy:

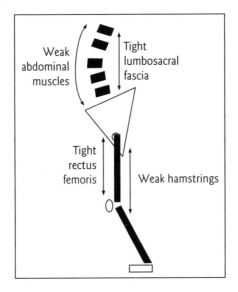

Figure 1.8

the spine being the straw, the muscles the cup around it? Push down on the rim of the cup with the flat palm of your hand, and the sides protect the straw. That's how the back works. Strong muscles help support the weight of the torso. Without their help, the spine and its many structures aren't protected. When you bend forward to hurl that bowling ball down the lane or simply to pick up a magazine, the weight shift puts more force on the vertebrae. Strong back muscles can contract and essentially neutralize that pressure. Weak muscles can't. Even taut abdominals pitch in, pushing back against the spine, helping to hold it stable and bearing some of its load (see figure 1.9).

Not only can trained muscles do more work, they can do it longer without fatiguing. Working out on a rowing machine is a good example. Rowing has the undeserved reputation of being a risky exercise for the back, not because it really is but because too many people think all you have to do is lower yourself onto the seat and start yanking away. Like any exercise, proper rowing form is

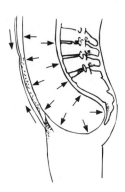

Figure 1.9

important, both for a good workout and to make sure your spine is loaded correctly. During the first few minutes that's easy. Fresh muscles hold your back just so. But as you get more and more tired, your form gets sloppy, and muscles that were not meant to help you pull the machine's "oars" have to get into the act. They won't thank you for it. And neither will your straw, er, spine.

As you will learn later in the book, the sports and activities in your life will dictate just which muscles most of your conditioning efforts must focus on. But before we get to that, you need to learn what can go wrong with your back.

Then you'll know exactly why we're doing what we're doing to keep it right.

...2...

Sciatica? No, That's Not It: Know What's *Really* Wrong with Your Back

Whether it's a household appliance, an automobile engine, or your back, nobody wants to go to a repair shop. So you try to follow good maintenance procedures, like changing the oil in your car as often as you're supposed to. And if you do have to bring it in for repairs, you need to find out exactly what went wrong and how to keep it from going wrong again.

With your back, to do this has been surprisingly difficult. Medicine and science have a frustrating way of lumping a large list of discomforts and pain under one umbrella word, as though sticking the label *sciatica* onto the ache in your lower spine and leg will help you understand what is happening. The label doesn't help, of course. In fact, it makes no more sense than telling a patient who's just hobbled in off the tennis court with a foot the size of a softball, "Well, I've examined your injury and I can now tell you that what you have here is called a swollen ankle."

However, while no physician would think of sending you away with a swollen ankle before telling you which ligaments you'd sprained, how much ice to apply and how often to apply it, which anti-inflammatories to take, what exercises you might do, and when you could expect to play doubles again, patients with back pain seldom receive anything nearly as helpful and specific. Instead you might very well hear, "A dull pain near your waist and radiating down your leg? Ah, yes. You have what we call 'sciatica.' " But to call the pain "sciatica" is not a diagnosis, certainly no more than "swollen ankle" is a diagnosis. In fact, sciatica is simply a symptom.

Sciatica, you see, is what you feel when something, somewhere, presses on the sciatic nerve—that complex web of fibers that run down through your spinal canal and join at the bottom of your spine before heading down the leg. And though you often feel the pain in your leg, the nerve is usually in trouble well upstream of that. But when sciatica is "diagnosed," *what* is doing the pressing, and *where,* is too often ignored. The source of your pain could be any one of a dozen things, but until a doctor knows for sure, planning treatment is about as scientific as throwing darts at a board. Maybe they stick, maybe they don't.

The key to a better understanding is in the very first step, and by that I mean asking the right questions at the beginning. And the way I learned that simple truth was to live through what began as one of the most boring mornings of my medical life and ended as one of the most important. I was in medical school, with a brilliant professor whose lectures wandered like a meandering stream. At first I thought he was slightly senile, but I soon realized that he was setting us up for one of the most important lessons we could ever learn.

The professor I am speaking of was J. Willis Hurst, M.D., a man who practiced medicine with the gift of a genius. He also taught the Clinical Methods course at Atlanta's Emory University School of Medicine. On opening day, he shuffled into class and began his lecture in a voice best described as country grit/third-generation tobacco farm drawl, and his clothes looked as if they hadn't been ironed since Reconstruction days. Like the rest of the medical students in Grady Auditorium that morning, I was ready to hang on every word. After all, this was *the* Dr. Hurst, the man who had been President Johnson's cardiologist and was now chairman of the Department of Medicine at Emory. We all hoped he would start us down the road to becoming real doctors by teaching the fine points of giving a thorough physical exam. And additionally, we all knew he was famous for telling students in a warm, paternal drawl that he would make sure we knew which end of the stethoscope goes into the ears.

Therefore, his opening remark was a shocker. "I'm sorry I'm late," he said, "but this morning while having breakfast I asked myself the question, how many Coca-Cola signs are there between my breakfast room and the Grady Auditorium?" Obviously this was not one of the burning questions keeping medical students up at night.

And the longer he spoke, the more odd his comments became. "I finished my Cheerios with no sugar, just a little bit of banana on the top for potassium, and skim milk. I eat very slowly, by the way, so I can enjoy my freshly squeezed orange juice to which I add a dash of grapefruit for a little tang. Then I got into my shirt, buttoned it, tied my tie, slipped on my white coat, lifted my briefcase, and got into my car. This morning I had to turn the key twice before it started."

Poor Dr. Hurst, we all thought as he rambled on like that for a good fifty minutes. Hurst detailed every move he'd made, from the time he sat down for breakfast to the moment he walked into the auditorium. Mind you, *every detail was recounted.*

Finally he said, "By now you must think J. Willis Hurst, M.D., is senile or on drugs. But I'm here to tell you that if I didn't ask myself the question this morning, how many Coca-Cola signs are there between my breakfast table and the Grady Auditorium? I wouldn't be able to stand here and tell you there are five. And *that* is what good medicine is all about!" he snapped. "If you don't ask the question, you will never know the answer. If you never wonder whether your patient has the heart murmur of aortic stenosis, you'll never hear it. If you never look for a medial collateral ligament tear in the knee, you'll never find it."

That concluded lecture number one, a lecture that has stayed with me all these years.

If a doctor doesn't look for the back pain of spinal stenosis, for example, he'll never find it. If he doesn't look for a leg-length discrepancy which could be throwing your gait off and causing your "back" problem, he'll never know if you have one. If he doesn't look for the arthritic, bony formation called an osteophyte on the vertebrae, he'll never be able to diagnose it. You'll never know what's wrong with your back. And chances are, even if you do improve at first with some painkillers and all-purpose exercises, you're not going to stay pain-free.

Truth is, most doctors aren't crazy about dealing with backs, and I'll tell you why. Patients with back problems often don't get better. They keep coming back with the same complaints even though the doctor has tried *everything* from exercise and physical therapy to bed rest and medication. So once a practitioner has determined the "category" of your problem, he'll put you into a "category" treatment and hope for the best. I say, "No, that's not it."

In my opinion, these generic diagnoses and all-purpose treatments don't help anyone get better, though statistics would seem to prove me wrong. There are statistics out there saying 50 percent of back patients recover within a week, 85 percent within one month, and more than 90 percent within two months. What the numbers don't tell you is that these figures hold true no matter what treatment the patients were given. And since it can't be that all therapies are equal, something else must be happening.

What is happening is this. A basketball player, for example, follows his doctor's generic treatment plan—whatever it is—and feels better immediately. So he goes right back to playing ball, but shortly there's that pain again. He returns to his doctor, gets better again, and repeats the cycle a couple of times before he decides to get another opinion. Still, every time he gets better, he's statistically counted as a recovery. Meanwhile, he's lost a lot of court time and put up with a lot of unnecessary discomfort.

What the basketball player needed all along was a treatment plan for his specific condition, one that would reinforce his back against the particular stresses of his sport. All pain has a way of vanishing if you stop doing what brought it on, but let's not confuse that with a *cure*. The problem is only waiting to come back, even though you're statistically "better" for the moment.

In this book, you're going to learn about many of the causes of back pain. Obviously I'm not going to try to diagnose your specific problem, nor should you diagnose it yourself. Leave that to a doctor. But when you do see a doctor, at least you're going to know which questions to ask. When you know more about your back, you'll know that "sciatica" is where the discussion should begin, not end. As an educated medical consumer, you'll want and appreciate a pinpoint diagnosis and a specific treatment plan.

But use your knowledge wisely, not like my back patient Ken, a twenty-eight-year-old accountant and probably the best educated medical consumer I've ever examined. Ken was also the hardest to treat.

Back patients sometimes come in carrying six-inch piles of old medical records from doctors past. But Ken, a distance runner who averaged sixty miles a week, had something far more enterprising: a six-inch stack of photocopies right out of medical textbooks. "Here, Doc," he said, shoving the material across my desk. "Read this, because that's what I have."

I resisted the temptation to ask why he hadn't bypassed my fee, as well as my expertise, and just gone into his own do-it-yourself therapy. "No, thanks," I said. "I've read my medical textbooks. What we're going to do is discuss your medical history, give you a physical exam, talk about what kind of pain you're in, and determine a treatment plan to get you better."

No dice. "Let's not waste time. I know what I have. Just tell me how to get better," he interrupted impatiently. When I finally convinced him that if he insisted on supplying the diagnosis he'd also have to supply the cure, he backed off and let me do my job.

The examination revealed that his conclusion was totally off. The so-called iliotibial band on the outside of his leg, which he was certain was causing all his trouble, was fine. His piriformis muscle, deep in the hip, was the problem. Often lumped in with—what else?—"sciatica," piriformis trouble takes intense and meticulously organized therapy. We'll discuss a little later in this chapter what actually happens, and you'll see that any patient who expects to get better needs to be dedicated to following instructions to the letter. Thanks to all his homework, Ken was willing to do just that. He knew what he had to do and why. He did it, and it paid off.

As you learn about what can go wrong with your back, like Ken, you will be more motivated to do what it takes to make the pain go away permanently. And you'll know just how to use the exercise program in this book to your advantage. Each routine is geared not only to the specific needs of your back but to your specific activities for a highly personalized program.

Keep the equation working to your advantage: the more you know about your back, the more you'll get out of this book, the better you'll feel, and, ultimately, the healthier your back will be. By learning about back anatomy in the previous chapter, you already know the language. Now let's talk about some of the most common causes of backaches and back pains.

So It Hurts. But Why?

As you will read in the following pages, any number of things can cause back pain. Some simply come from the way your body is put together—your biomechanics. Do you habitually sit with your back hunched forward? Yes, that can do it. So can running with your foot turned just the slightest bit inward. So can going on lots of long bike rides when your hips aren't loose and flexible.

The voluntary mistakes are easily fixed: you don't make them anymore. If hunching or slouching is just laziness or muscle weakness, get smart, get in shape, and get rid of your back trouble. But with a genetic predisposition, life's not going to be simple. If your father or mother has a foot that rolls inward when he or she walks, chances are you will too. But recognizing the problem is half the battle, since it helps you find a solution—exercises, or perhaps shoe inserts if warranted—to offset your imbalances and keep your spine and its muscles happy.

Probably the most feared cause of back trouble is trauma, when there's been actual damage to one of the spine's structures. The damage could be a pulled muscle or a bulging disk, and the trouble could happen suddenly when your Great Dane sees a comely dalmatian across the street and decides to take you and your back muscles with him *right now.* Or it could happen little by little as the disks are worn down by the jarring of hundreds of weekly sprints up and down the basketball court. In trauma cases, by the way, the pain is usually constant and stays the same regardless of how you're sitting, standing, or moving.

To make things more interesting yet, you can have a genetic susceptibility to what seem like sudden traumas. For example, degenerated disks, which are more easily damaged, may run in your family.

Occasionally back pain has nothing to do with your back. A kidney infection feels a lot like a bad back. So can ulcers, urinary tract infections, and a lot of less common conditions, like pelvic inflammatory disease, tubal pregnancy, prostatitis, pancreatitis, and even gout, which most people think settles in the lower leg. And there are more. The gravest, of course, is when the pain comes from a tumor located near or even on the spine. Unless there's a reason to do otherwise, your doctor will understandably begin looking at your back as the source of your back pain. But if nothing turns up after careful investigation, and if the pain persists for more than a few weeks, you should probably begin looking for answers outside the back.

Curve Causes: The Trouble with Lordosis, Kyphosis, and Scoliosis

In the last chapter we admired the back's elegant "S" curve and the way it helps absorb shock and insures that the weight of the torso is well distributed among the vertebrae. But too much curve, we also said, is not a good thing. Lordosis, the exaggeration of the back's lumbar curve, kyphosis, the exaggeration of the back's thoracic (upper back) curve, and scoliosis, a mild or severe deformity in which the spine curves out to the side, are all shifts in the "S" that can stress the spine (see figure 2.1). One possible consequence of lordosis—which can come simply from poor posture or even from lugging around an excessive load in the front of the body, such as during pregnancy or, less romantic, after the growth of a beer belly—is a form of what we call spinal stenosis. The tilt puts pressure on the

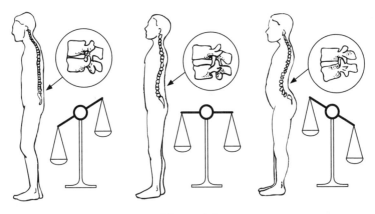

Figure 2.1

back part of the vertebrae, narrowing the spinal canal that runs through them and possibly even pinching the spinal cord.

Kyphosis, by contrast, loads the front of the vertebrae, so this time it's the disk that gets the squeeze. Squeezed too long and too hard, it may begin to bulge, which is sometimes the prelude to a rupture. Kyphosis can come simply from standing or sitting stoop-shouldered. It can also be a by-product of osteoporosis, the bone-thinning disease that affects more women than men, especially after menopause, and causes the spine to round forward.

Scoliosis, when the spine curves to one side or the other, is serious enough and starts early enough in life that most doctors examining schoolchildren know to screen for it. Caught early, scoliosis can be treated with a brace. Adults who missed out may be prone to back pain primarily because the muscles of any spine that's out of alignment must labor harder to keep the body balanced. Vertebrae, too, can bear a heavy burden. The exaggerated curve can also result in the pinching of some nerves, radiating pain to wide areas of the back. Although scoliosis is usually congenital and obvious early in life, adults can actually develop it as their disks degenerate.

And there's even a variation of kyphosis that some people call "butterflier's back," since the rounding of the upper spine in that swim stroke looks just like it. You'll sometimes also hear it called Scheuermann's disease, but I don't consider it a disease. This variation of kyphosis is really a growth disturbance of the vertebral bodies as they're developing, and it affects mostly children and adolescents. Rounding your back forward hurts, which means the last thing people with "butterflier's back" should do is the butterfly stroke. As with scoliosis, when the problem is addressed in youngsters, the child stands an excellent chance of full recovery. But anyone who makes it to adulthood without having the exaggerated curve corrected will have to live with it—and possibly the back pain that comes with it.

Vertebrae Trouble: The Pain of Spondylolysis and Spondylolisthesis

In the last chapter we described the vertebrae as the building blocks of the spine, the sturdy, cleverly designed stacked structures of bone that give us shape. And they do. But while the design is clever, it is not perfect. There are weak spots and flaws that too often don't stay hidden.

A football lineman and an adolescent gymnast, for example, may not seem to have much in common when it comes to courting vertebrae trouble. But they do. Both are candidates for the tongue-twisting condition called *spondylolysis,* a stress fracture in the back portion of the vertebra, specifically in the arched area attached to the bony processes (see figure 2.2). This area of bone, called the pars interarticularis, is actually comparatively weak and unable to withstand a whole lot of pressure, especially the kind it gets when the back is stretched into an excessive arch, a condition we call "hyperextended." Gymnasts and skaters who go into extreme back bends, football players who push up and

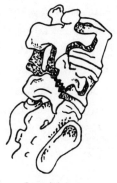

Spondylolysis

Figure 2.2

out from a crouched position on the line, long jumpers who arch their backs over the pit—all are candidates. But you don't have to be a football player or gymnast to suffer from this malady. One good hyperextension on a vertebra that can't handle it will bring the condition on.

While hyperextension may trigger spondylolysis, other motions, mostly athletic, can do it too. A collision can fracture the back of the vertebra, as many football linemen can tell you. So can repetitive jumping as in gymnastics, or unremitting pounding such as long-distance runners' bodies often experience. The heavy weights pumped by a bodybuilder, and even the relatively lighter ones of a hiker's backpack, can often be enough, as are the twisting moves of hard-played racquet sports, softball, and golf, and even subtler arching moves in rowing, volleyball, and basketball.

So it's not surprising that athletes are probably at greater risk for spondylolysis. According to a study published in the early 1990s in the *Physician and Sports Medicine,* only 5 percent of spondylolysis sufferers come from the general population. Divers, weight lifters, wrestlers, gymnasts, and track and field athletes make up the rest. It's one of the few back pain advantages the couch potato can claim.

Spondylolisthesis, even harder to pronounce, is spondylolysis put into motion (see figure 2.3). If the pars interarticularis begins to separate at the stress fracture, the whole vertebra can come sliding forward, throwing the spinal column out of whack. If the bone slides just beyond 25 percent, it's usually time for surgery to fuse it back into place.

Though both conditions sound grave, ordinarily neither by itself causes back pain. But both have the potential to make the area unstable, and when that happens, the odds go up that some part of the vertebra will rub against a nerve. And you know by now what that does. Instability can also put a strain on the ligaments and muscles, making them work overtime. Overworked muscles usually let you know it, too.

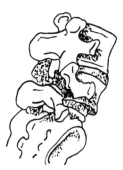

Spondylolisthesis

Figure 2.3

Spinal Stenosis: The Too-Tight Canal

The vertebrae are essentially to blame for spinal stenosis. The spinal canal ought to be the perfect protective tube for the body's lifeline, with the vertebrae stacked one on top of another and the hole in each creating a tunnel that comfortably encircles and protects the spinal cord and nerves. Yet that very same protector can narrow and rub against the things it's supposed to protect. That turnabout is called *spinal stenosis*.

Some people are born with a stingy canal, but the narrowing of the canal can also come on later in life. When a disk begins to lose water in the natural aging process, for example, it can actually cause the foramen—the opening in the vertebra that encircles the cord—to narrow. Osteoarthritis, a condition that affects the tri-joint complex, can also cause the foramen to close in.

Whatever the cause, spinal stenosis hurts. It can be one of the many causes behind numbness and tingling in the legs, symptoms we loosely call "sciatica" if the nerve being rubbed happens to be the sciatic nerve.

Step one for anyone with the condition is to avoid *all* extreme bending, which is the last thing that occurs to most of us. It had certainly never occurred to Janet, the college professor having spasms in her lower back and sciatic pain down her leg. The pain was beginning to interfere with her teaching. She had already begun strapping on a lumbar support during her daily railroad commute, and going to a gym to strengthen her abdominal and back muscles. Good thinking on the face of it, but bad medicine. Janet was doing full sit-ups as part of the basic six exercises she'd read about in one back article after another. She was also cranking out a full range-of-motion movement on back extension and flexion machines—back-bending movements every single one—and all of that flexing and extending was squeezing her spinal cord even more. Instead she should have been doing abdominal crunches rather than sit-ups, and less range of motion on the back extension machine. When Janet made these changes, she was once again a pain-free professor.

Other common "remedies" can make spinal stenosis worse. Heat, for instance. Every part of the body exposed to heat will swell, and this includes the soft tissues surrounding the spinal cord. As an example, if you have spinal stenosis and you sit in a whirlpool, then go out and take an aerobics class, the consequence is that your swollen nerves are far more likely to end up rubbing against their narrowed casing. That's why we call the pain that comes on this way "spa back."

Much to the dismay of the sufferer, people with spinal stenosis have to learn to take cooler showers and stay out of steamy whirlpools and hot tubs. And they have to watch out for physical therapists offering hot packs to warm up their patients' muscles before helping them stretch. The purpose of warm-up, naturally, is to soften the muscles into warm taffy so that they will stretch more easily; a hot pack is a passive way of achieving that. Under normal circumstances this is a perfectly good way to go about it. Hot packs also allow a therapist to work on more than one patient at a time. But a better procedure, especially for a patient with spinal stenosis, is to use active warm-up, otherwise known as exercise. Get on a stationary bicycle and pedal for five minutes, just breaking a sweat, and you'll increase your temperature half a degree and warm your muscles entirely—not just the outside, which is what a hot pack does.

Disk Risks: Degeneration, Herniation, and Bulges

In the last chapter I described disks as the cushions between the vertebral bodies. You now know that the disk is made up of a hardish outer shell called the annulus fibrosus and a soft, gelatinous center called the nucleus pulposus. And you know that despite the seemingly humble appearance of this "jelly donut," it is intricate, complex, and frequently the source of back pain.

The trouble usually begins when the disk's shell and its contents begin to degenerate (see figure 2.4). Disks may degenerate naturally—that is, flatten and lose some of their shock-absorbing power—as the body ages. For one thing, older bodies retain less water, so like our other parts, the H_2O-absorbing molecules (proteoglycans) in the disk's nucleus become less imbibed. The disk, as a result, dehydrates, deflating like an old balloon. Degeneration also occurs because the disks help carry a

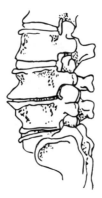

Figure 2.4

heavy load, the weight of your torso. Over time, body weight simply wears them down.

Biomechanics figures into the degeneration of disks too, because every movement you make increases the load on your spine, so the disks of a highly active person are subject to more pressure. Some movements, of course, add more stress than others, like lifting weights or running seventy miles a week. In fact, though the repetitive jarring of your feet hitting the pavement day after day may not produce any effects for years—at least nothing you'd notice—the annulus layers may slowly begin to tear, weakening the outer layer until, finally, there's a bulge or herniation.

Though not all at once, rotational movement can also put stress on disks. Obviously you don't have a perfectly healthy annulus fibrosus one minute, then swing a golf club and *bam,* it's ruptured. No, the breakdown is much subtler and harder to see coming. You really need to rotate again and again and again, and finally the annulus fibrosus of a disk begins to break down. Twist a paper straw in one direction enough times and the paper fibers begin to fray; and so it is with the annulus. With enough twisting, the gelatinous middle will ooze into the weakened-wall area and push against the frail tissue to create a bulge. Twist hard enough and the annulus may burst, spilling its contents. At this unhappy moment you've herniated—or blown—a disk.

It's tempting to think that only a dramatic strain can produce so dramatic a result. I wish that were so. Truth is, even everyday moves like lifting a heavy box without bending your knees, which forces your back to act as a lever, is often all it takes if the disk is already weakened. That one sneeze, the one bad move, can cause the gelatinous middle to push right out of the disk.

But instead of understanding that it's a weakness that has been coming on by degrees and that some mundane movement finally brought into the open, we persist in thinking some major mistake we made caused this injury all at once. By the time Joey arrived in my office he had, like most patients, assigned full blame to himself for his troubles. A thirty-eight-year-old writer on his way back from a business trip one winter Sunday, he was in a hurry to get home to watch a Giants game. No sooner was the plane at the gate than Joey was on his feet and reaching for his luggage in the overhead compartment. Suddenly a woman in fear of missing her connection rushed down the aisle toward him. Joey jumped onto his toes and simultaneously yanked his heavy garment bag out of the overhead compartment, just as she barreled into him, throwing him wildly off balance. An hour later Joey could barely walk into his apartment. Pain shot through the sciatic nerve in his leg down to his big toe. He watched the game flat on his back, was pumped up with anti-inflammatories, and wondered what he'd done wrong.

Joey had blown a disk. But it wasn't entirely his fault. Had he stood straight while lifting his suitcase directly over his head with no sideways body blows, nothing would have gone wrong—at least that time—because the "S" curve in his back could have distributed the bag's weight evenly among his disks and vertebrae. But because he was on tiptoe, his arms were raised, and he was bent at the waist to get out of the lady's way, he was out of optimal position for so heavy a load. His disk probably had plenty of microtears in it all along, but the blow finally pushed it over the edge. "If only I hadn't tried to be a nice guy, it would never have happened," he groaned. That's how it seemed, but that's not how it was. Chivalry, or whatever, didn't do it all at once. Nature did it, little by little.

Degeneration, bulges, herniation—however a disk becomes flawed, it usually ends up causing you pain. When it degenerates, the vertebrae it separates move closer together so there's less movement possible between them, and the whole tri-joint complex gets thrown off. As the disk flattens, the vertebra on top of it shifts downward, as do the facet joints attached to it. This not only disrupts their alignment, decreasing their ability to move well, but it may also narrow the openings the nerves run through. The result: bone rubs on nerve, and nerve hurts.

It's no picnic when a disk bulges or herniates. Bending forward (which we all do a hundred times a day without thinking) squeezes the front of our disks and sends the soft center toward the back, which is why bulges generally occur toward the posterior of the vertebrae—right where they can easily press on a nerve. Herniations, likewise, usually end up spilling back into the spinal canal, where the gelatinous substance not only presses on but also chemically irritates the nerves.

Pain, for sure. But pain *where*? That's one of the few exact things about diagnosing back trouble. The location of the pain usually tells me which disk is your problem. If it's a lumbar disk, you're likely to have discomfort in your lower back or down your leg, called "referred pain"—sciatica. When the troubled disk is cervical, you feel the pain in your neck, shoulders, arms, or hands. Precisely pinpointing the hurt can tell us exactly which disk it is. If sciatic pain radiates through the front of the thigh, for example, it's a good bet that disk L4-5 is causing the trouble.

Unfortunately, the problem may not necessarily stop there. A painful nerve can stir up still more trouble by sending a muscle into spasm. Alerted to the unhappy nerve or even just the change in spinal alignment, the vigilant but not always wise body sends the muscles that support the back into action to help out. Whether or not the muscles are up to the job, they keep on trying, eventually growing exhausted and coming down with a muscle's version of the hiccups—involuntary and sharp contractions. So you hurt even more.

A disk that has degenerated, bulged, or herniated will never regain its youth. That's the bad news. The good news is that that may not necessarily be such bad news. Sometimes the fingerlike bulge touching the nerve eventually dissolves all by itself. A good stretching and strengthening program can often rout the pain and let you get back to whatever you were doing—with care. Remember: the affected area is weak and always will be, so you'll need to take some precautions when you do get back into action. A swimmer might have to give up the butterfly stroke and stay with freestyle, for example.

The Pain in the Neck Nobody Needs

Disk problems can happen near the neck (the cervical region) just as they can lower down. The spaces for the nerves grow smaller, causing irritation and "referred pain" down the arm or in the shoulder blade. But thankfully, this pain can almost always be cured without surgery. In fact, relieving pressure on the nerve due to a herniation is usually as easy as gently separating the vertebrae with the help of a neck traction device that's no more complicated than a bag full of water, a chin strap, and a rope to connect the two that you can hang over a door.

To achieve this, your cervical spine needs a constant, gentle upward tug to produce what I like to call the "Slinky effect," named for the child's springlike toy that opens and spreads as you pull on its ends. Think of what happens when you tug on a spring and the coils separate from each other. That's how your vertebrae behave when you sit on a chair and put on a chin strap that's connected over a pulley to a water-filled bag. The upward tug separates the vertebrae by stretching your spine, freeing the nerve. But the therapy requires patience. During the first half hour, your muscles try to fight back and nothing gets done. Eventually they give up and relax, and your vertebrae start to benefit. A one-hour sitting is normal.

The cervical vertebrae are more delicate than the ones beneath them and are well worth protecting, as any genuine victim of automotive whiplash can tell you. A minor rear-end automobile collision is usually enough to do the damage, though any mishap that either whips your head back and forth or sends a strong shock straight down your back can give you cervical trouble, no matter what your age. Recently a fifteen-year-old football player came in with his mother, who didn't think he should still be having neck pain three days after an especially rough tackle. His neck had bothered him immediately, but his coach's advice had been to apply ice and "get back in there." The coach's theory was, don't worry about it. If it feels worse, go to a doctor.

And here he was. I asked him why he hadn't gone to an emergency room right away. "My arms didn't hurt, my legs didn't hurt, and I could walk fine. So I didn't worry," was his logical reply. But he had been wrong. A simple X ray showed a compression fracture at C4.

Had he known how his "S" curve works, we might never have needed our conversation, because the curve in his neck and yours can normally deflect the pressure of most reasonable impact. But when the neck is flexed, as it is when your chin is down, the curve is lost. The cervical spine becomes a straight column, not a curved spring, so there's no shock-absorbing slope to soften the blow and it compresses everything in its path. That can spell fracture, as it had with our fifteen-year-old (see figure 2.5). If only he had kept his chin up even slightly as he went for the tackle, we'd probably never have met.

Front impact can also fracture cervical vertebrae. A tackle who takes a hit in the face head-on is putting the back of his cervical vertebrae to the test, since that's where the force ends up. The supporting muscles and ligaments may help soften the blow and avoid a fracture, but they develop problems of their own. If the force is great enough, the ligaments get yanked and you've got a classic case of whiplash.

My patient probably won't play again until he is seventeen, but it could have been worse. Untreated fractures

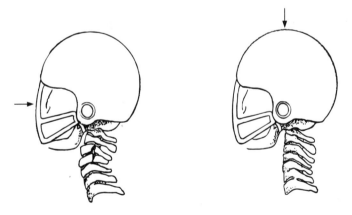

Figure 2.5

can do spinal cord damage we don't even want to talk about here. The lesson is: If you have neck pain after an impact, even with no serious symptoms, such as pain in the arms and legs, get thee to an X-ray machine.

Back Joints Get Arthritis Too

Will you develop osteoarthritis, and if so, how soon? It varies in all of us and is largely genetic. A look at your family history will usually give you an accurate preview.

In your back, osteoarthritis can affect the tri-joint complex—facet joints and disk—causing the whole thing to wear down and in the process tipping the precise balance of the vertebrae. If the facet joints get out of alignment, thrown off, for example, by the bony deposits of osteoarthritis (remember that gliding and aligning are the job of the joints), the spine starts to get unstable and the muscles trying to support it have to labor harder to keep it balanced. On top of that, the gliding surfaces of the facet joints have nerves of their own, which pick up this friction as pain.

At the same time, the spaces that encircle the nerves of the spinal cord can become narrowed, increasing even more the risk of friction and irritation.

Finally, the vertebrae could settle closer together, possibly enough to limit your ability to bend forward or backward.

Osteoarthritis can also help trigger the formation of osteophytes, tiny bone formations that the body creates as it works futilely to keep everything aligned. While they can and sometimes do work, keeping the facet joints in line and allowing free movement to continue, these small bone formations can also inadvertently press on a nerve. Now you've got pain in one place from trying to avoid it in another. Nature doesn't always know best.

Facet Syndrome

A few years ago, a study that surprised a lot of doctors seemed to indicate that facet joints are at the root of the trouble for nearly eight out of ten back patients. Sounds high to me, but it does show that these gliding joints have plenty of opportunity for mischief. We usually call the facet joint defect "facet syndrome," restricted motion and off-balance alignment that upsets the neatly stacked vertebrae and puts the nerves at risk. Facet joint trouble can even indirectly cause sciatic pain as the muscles around the spine go into spasm from all of that heroic balancing work.

Arthritis is one thing that can make a good gliding joint go bad. Trauma is another, like crashing down on the field in a soccer game or taking a header on an icy sidewalk, which can inflame the fibrous capsule containing the joint. Facet damage can also occur gradually as the thinning disk (facet joints' partner in the tri-joint complex) permits the joints' surfaces to rub and grow rough.

Sometimes, though, the joints aren't damaged at all, they've just slipped off line. One of the most satisfying things a chiropractor can do for you is slip them back into place, releasing any trapped nerves and eliminating your pain, just like that.

Muscle Strains and Ligament Sprains

Again and again I've talked about how the muscles in the back are crucial to the support and protection of the spine. For that reason alone you need to keep them well conditioned. But keeping them in shape will also help them weather stress and strain; and when I tell you that most back problems are actually caused by muscles that are not strong or supple enough to do their job, you can see how useful good ones can be.

Just ask Sandra, a twenty-eight-year-old second-grade teacher who spends weekdays running after her kids and weekends playing doubles tennis with her husband. On a summer Sunday not long ago, Sandra was in the middle of a tight, take-no-prisoners match when she cocked her arm back to power a serve and instead crumpled to the court, grabbing at the pain in her lower back. Sandra's husband dived for his cellular phone, and within minutes I was on my way to meet them at the emergency room. The suddenness and the sharpness of the pain terrified Sandra. "Oh my god," she cried. "I blew a disk. Please, I don't want surgery." I calmed her, cautioning that one thing you never do with the back is jump to conclusions.

So we took X rays and found that Sandra hadn't blown a disk at all. It was a simple muscle pull that felt like something far more serious. And the therapy was as plain and effective as it gets: ice treatments, a few days of rest, then an exercise program to strengthen that muscle and some of the others it works with. Sandra was back on the courts in two weeks as if nothing had happened. The only scary part about her back "condition" was what she had imagined might have happened.

Back muscles are susceptible to injury primarily because they work so diligently, with very little time off. Even when you're just standing still, the postural muscles are keeping you stable. And they work harder yet when you're sitting. They labor hardest of all, naturally, when you're active, controlling every move your back makes, from opening a cabinet to throwing a softball.

"Taking it easy" isn't enough to protect them, either. I don't care if pulling on the refrigerator door is as tough as life gets for your back muscles, you can strain them if they're not primed to do even that modest amount of work. That's why flexibility is so important. Your back muscles are like rubber bands attached to the vertebrae. When they're too tight, a sudden move can cause them to snap— not literally, of course, just enough to tear some tissues. What's more, tight muscles tug on the spine, potentially throwing the vertebrae out of alignment. The result: pain from the vertebrae and stiffness from the tight tissues.

Once we get your conditioning program under way, you'll see that the muscles don't even have to be in your back to cause back pain. For example, the hamstrings in the back of your legs and the quadriceps in the front may seem far removed from your spine, but they are connected to muscles that in turn are attached to your spine. So if either leg muscle is tight, it will pull on the back muscle, which will pass the tension right along to the spine. Your back muscles are like a delicately balanced triangle, with the spine, hamstrings, and quads all applying tension. If one side is too tight, the triangle tips, throwing the other sides off balance.

Obviously muscle strain can happen in an instant. It can also come on gradually. If you have poor posture—say you slump when you sit or you let your abdomen stick out when you stand—your muscles have to work extra hard to keep you stable. Eventually they're going to feel the strain. Think of how stiff and sore your neck gets when you use it to wedge the phone onto your shoulder so that your hands will be free to write a message. The next step for over-worked muscles is usually a continued state of contraction, also known as spasm.

Sprains—more properly called ligament strains—can also start muscle spasming. Your back's ligaments, as we said in chapter 1, act as a sort of support stocking for the vertebrae. Back ligaments are a lot like the ones in your ankles, and just like the ligaments in your ankles, which you can sprain if you're not careful, back ligaments heal. That often comes as a nice surprise to patients who fear that a "sprained back" diagnosis is a preamble to some-thing medically long, complicated, scary, and expensive. It certainly needn't be. The immediate pain comes from the ligaments themselves, which are equipped with nerve end-ings to warn when something's wrong. What happens next is that the particular part of the body the ligament used to support must now be held in place by nearby muscles, which can get overworked and go into spasm. And have more pain. The spasms may even irritate a nerve that goes down your leg, and—guess what? You've got "sciatica." But now you know that's not really it.

Coming Up Short:
Leg-Length Discrepancies

Sometimes the key to your "back" problem is all the way down at the bottom of your feet. And as Dr. J. Willis Hurst warned his students that morning, "If you don't look for it, you'll never find it."

For example, your legs might be exactly the same length physically, but they may function differently. Let me explain. Leg-length discrepancies, which by the way are the most common source of back pain among runners (remember Tony, whose story I told earlier?), can of course be anatomical. Many people are born this way, the body rarely being the perfectly symmetrical work of art we like to think it is. Or the discrepancy can be functional, meaning the legs measure the same, but something about the way you move makes one leg *act* shorter than the other. As an example, when you walk or run, you might turn one foot outward (called supinating) or inward (called pronating, most common among flat-footed folk). That little twist effectively lengthens the leg every time it hits the ground. If you don't move around much, a leg-length discrepancy might escape notice for a lifetime. But active people, and especially those who run, can develop back problems from even a tiny imbalance.

Anatomical or functional, a leg-length discrepancy will knock your muscles out of alignment just as surely as pulling a toy building block from the bottom of a child's tower will make it tilt. But unlike a toy tower, the body responds, working to compensate for the imbalance. The spine curves to the side, one hip rides up, one shoulder pulls down. These little adjustments not only put pressure on the vertebrae and stress on the ligaments, they can also strain muscles, which are already working hard to keep things stable.

Frankly, I am always delighted to discover that a back patient has a leg-length discrepancy, because it's so easy to fix. A simple heel lift in the shoe or an orthotic insert to correct pronation does away with the problem. Orthotics, by the way, have to fit just so, or you'll exchange an aggravating back for aggravated feet.

The Vicious Pain Cycle: Trigger Points

But what about pain that just never goes away, yet seems to have no physical cause? Are there backs that are just meant to hurt this way? No. But there are some backs that have more "trigger points" than others. And when trigger points get going, they make sure your discomfort never ends.

To understand what happens, let's review how the body responds to pain. When you touch the flame of a match or candle, little receptors in your finger fire off a message to the spinal cord telling it what a stupid thing you've done. The spinal cord then shoots an electrical message back to the muscles of the finger, telling them to contract and get away from that painful flame. At the same time it sends a message up to the brain that says, "Ouch!" But you don't even feel the ouch until your finger has already been pulled away.

In the back it goes something like this: You pull a muscle and, responding to the strain, it goes into spasm. As it contracts, it presses down on a nerve, which sends an SOS to the spinal cord. "Ouch! There's pain over here!" So the spinal cord, not knowing all the details, sends a directive back to the muscle saying, "Better contract and get away from that pain!" And so it all starts again—a closed loop of self-inflicted discomfort. Sometimes an ice massage can break the cycle, sometimes anti-inflammatories can do the trick. Or you may need to get a deep-tissue massage or have electrogalvanic stimulation treatments (the closest thing we have today to Hippocrates's electric eel) to disrupt the electrical circle that's perpetuating the cycle.

You can have more than one trigger point. Lots more. John, a forty-eight-year-old banker and runner who came to see me for back pain he'd been struggling with for more than two years, turned out to have seventeen trigger points! At first he didn't believe he had any. All he had done was fall on the basketball court, he said, and he must have thrown something out way back then. The CAT scan and MRI he brought to our first appointment showed essentially nothing. Even his disks were in great shape.

The trigger points were the whole problem. I could feel them—knotty little balls in the muscles—so I sent him to physical therapy for electrogalvanic stimulation to break the vicious cycle. Once he understood what we needed to do, he was as compulsive about therapy as he had been about running. In less than a month, the cycle was over and John was pain-free for the first time in two years.

That True Pain in the Butt:
Piriformis Syndrome

While we're on the subject of pain cycles, there's a muscle down in your butt, the piriformis, that's likely to try the same kind of trick. Remember Ken, the patient with the huge stack of photocopies from medical textbooks and the do-it-yourself diagnosis, earlier in this chapter? He found out about piriformis the hard way. And wonder of wonders, piriformis is *another* pain that usually gets the "sciatica" label pasted on it. Here's why.

The problem starts as a dull ache in the middle of one buttock, especially sharp if you run on it and worse yet going up hills or walking up stairs. It's easy to tar it with the low-back-pain brush, not so easy to suspect the piriformis, one of the muscles deep in the rear of the pelvis. The piriformis helps turn your leg outward and runs alongside, and occasionally surrounds, the sciatic nerve. Like any muscle, it can be overused and go into spasm, something runners and ballet dancers know particularly well. Even tight hamstring muscles, prolonged sitting, or anything that twists the area can irritate the piriformis.

When that happens—and especially when the nearby sciatic nerve becomes involved—the pain is dull, constant, and seemingly permanent. Diagnosis is not difficult. One or two simple exercises can pinpoint the trouble, and trained fingers can actually feel down to and sense the spasming muscle.

But diagnosis is only the beginning and therapy is far from simple. Because the muscle is so deep and the spasm so hard to break, we usually need to gang up several therapies besides exercise, including a specialized technique called transverse frictional massage, electrogalvanic stimulation, ice, and ultrasound. But when the artillery is heavy and the logistics are right, the pain does go.

• • •

Ow! you say. If all that can happen to my back, what chance do I have of being pain-free? Well, you could be one of the lucky ones who never has trouble, especially if you work on your potential problems before they get to work on you. A healthy, well-maintained back is obviously everyone's best defense. But it's also important to know that there are therapies and treatments that address each of these problems. Let me tell you next what these treatments and remedies are. And then let's talk about exactly what you can do so you never need them, or, if it's too late for that, so you'll never need them again.

...**3**...

Job One: Getting a Pain-Free Back

Chances are, you picked up this book for the same reasons you'd buy a computer virus program. Either your common sense said the odds of trouble are growing all the time and you want to be ready when it strikes, or it's already too late and you need help fixing the problem. Well, I can't tell you anything about your hard drive, but if it's your spine that's bothering you, I can assure you there's plenty that can and should be done. Even if you've just had some seemingly minor telltale warnings—a mysterious pain that vanished as inexplicably as it came—there are steps you can take to keep it from troubling you again.

I would have an easy job as a back doctor if all I had to think about was healthy backs. But life is neither that rosy nor that fair. So as your back book doc, I want to first discuss what to do if you develop back pain and what options you'll have for treating it. Then, once you're on the way to having that strong back, you can start the program in part II of this book, a program that will teach you how to enjoy a healthy, pain-free back.

In an Accident, Every Minute Counts

First, we need to decide how much time you've got to plan your treatment. If you've had an accident, the answer is, not much. And by accident, I don't mean something as common as reaching awkwardly up into the overhead airplane locker and unleashing a spasming muscle. I mean getting rear-ended in your car. Or spinning your bike wheels out from underneath you. Or taking a header on the ice with your arms full of groceries. Accidents such as these are called "trauma," because they demand immediate attention.

Warning number one: if it hurts too much to move, *don't move.* Let the emergency medical technicians who will help you to the hospital put you on a back board to get you there. If there's any chance you've fractured or broken a bone in your back, lying flat and motionless on the board will keep your spine stable so you don't risk damaging delicate nerves that may be in harm's way. A little helpless embarrassment (or feeling silly about it) could conceivably prevent a limb from becoming paralyzed later.

Warning number two: don't be a hero, confident that "I can walk around just fine, thanks, so you EMTs be on your way," or "I'll just drive myself to the doctor in the morning after I get the kids to school." There are so-called stable fractures, momentarily willing to remain in place but really quite unstable if they're mechanically aggravated by something even as gentle as walking.

This is not alarmist doctor talk. I've actually seen several cases where patients stepped out of their cars after an accident, found they could get around rather nicely, and refused to be taken in on a back board for X rays. Later, having partially lost the use of a limb, they regretted their misplaced stoicism. *Be safe.* Accept the help that is offered and go for X rays if needed.

If you have suffered a back break or fracture, don't think it means you've seen the last of sports and other physically demanding pastimes. Dr. Michael Neuwirth knows. He was the spinal surgeon in charge of singer Gloria Estefan's case, after she broke her back in a bus accident. Although she required surgery, she is once again performing with gusto, prancing and dancing and exploding all over the stage with the musical energy that has always propelled her career. And she's by no means a surgical anomaly. Quarterback Joe Montana, New York Giants offensive tackle John ("Jumbo") Elliot, and the Boston Celtics' Larry Bird—to do just a little back surgery name-dropping—have all required back operations of one sort or another, and have bounced back to the kind of bone-bruising play that few nonprofessional athletes ever pursue. So a broken back, literally speaking, doesn't automatically mean you'll be living the rest of your life on the sidelines, and good back surgery will not leave you on the sidelines, either.

When Bad Backs Are No Accident

But mercifully, car wrecks and crushing tackles don't happen to most of us. What does happen is that one day you just wake up and, *Ow!*, what's *that* in my back? Or you straighten up after lowering Sally, the golden Labrador, into the washtub and wonder if that sudden pain you've never felt before will let you bend back over to actually give her a bath. Strange. You've washed Sally dozens of times without anything like this happening.

Then we all ask the very same questions: What did I do wrong? What do I do now? And how quickly do I need to do it?

While it is important to have a complete diagnosis so you can then engage in a complete treatment plan—as I'll never tire of saying—there's probably no need to rush off to the hospital. If you must, you can wait the weekend before getting in to see your physician.

What to do in the meantime? Probably not what you think. If moving around is an effort, then of course lie down. But be careful. Twenty-four to thirty-six hours of bed rest is very likely all you'll need to get back to something like your normal routine, although you should expect some residual pain and stiffness. If that amount of time is not long enough to make a noticeable difference, there are good reasons to get up anyway.

If you stay in bed any longer than thirty-six hours, the muscles that support the back become progressively weaker. While your back muscles in this situation are weakening, your disks are taking advantage of the breather to soak up or "imbibe" water, as I mentioned earlier in the book. And though normally well hydrated, plump disks help keep a back healthy, suddenly heavy, drinking disks do not. In fact, they can be dangerous if there's any chance you have a herniation in one of them. Stay in bed for a week with the disks continuing to absorb water, and those proteoglycans I discussed in chapter 2 will drink up so much that the disks will grow extra puffy. When you finally stand up and put weight on them, any leakage from the center—the herniation—will have that much more fluid to spill, possibly pushing out with greater force right onto the painful nerve.

So do stay in bed just long enough to let things calm down, and do relax while you're at it. The tension of anxiety not only gets you nowhere, it can actually make things worse if part of your problem is a muscle so tense that it's already in spasm.

Besides, you will have too many constructive things to do to just lie around worrying. Take a Ziploc freezer bag, fill it with ice and water, and apply it to the painful area in your back for twenty minutes at least four times a day to soothe the nerve. The water you'll add to the ice raises the temperature of the mixture to thirty-two degrees Fahrenheit so you can apply it directly to the skin and not be afraid of getting freezer burn.

Then, since your pain is probably originating in an inflamed area around a nerve somewhere, calm it down even more with an over-the-counter medication like acetaminophen (Tylenol), aspirin, ibuprofen (Advil, Nuprin), or naproxen (Aleve). Choose whichever one you know agrees with you. I have no special preference. For now, unless you've already been advised otherwise by your doctor, stay away from anything stronger you may have in the medicine cabinet.

After thirty-six hours of bed rest, start moving—but *slowly, gently,* very conservatively. Maybe walk around the block once, and call it a day. It's important not to overdo any movement. Even mild exercise like this is recommended only to gently wake up your back muscles until you get to the root of your problem.

The doctor is your next stop—that is, unless you've also noticed any of the following symptoms, in which case you should already have seen a doctor. If you suddenly find you're having trouble controlling your urine or your bowel movements, or if your legs feel like they've become weak or numb and just don't want to do what you want them to, throw the one-step-at-a-time approach I've just offered right out the window. Get to the doctor as early as you possibly can, because a nerve may not be just irritated, it may be in real danger. Prompt action can make a difference.

And if your day and a half of bed rest seems like a perfect time to lie back and light up, please listen to what I have to say. Granted, you've probably made your decision to smoke knowing the health risks you're taking, so I won't bore you with yet another sermon on that subject. But now, something else is at work in your body that you may not have heard about.

Researchers now know that nicotine constricts your blood vessels, a process that also decreases the blood supply to anything that's injured. Researchers also know that statistical studies prove that obesity, psychological problems, *and smoking* boost your chances of back problems. One study, in fact, shows smokers with a low back pain risk of up to two and one-half times greater than that of non-smokers. Another study looked at identical twins whose only fundamental health difference was that one smoked and the other didn't. It was determined that the twin who smoked was more likely to come down with degenerative changes in the spine. So if you smoke and you're having back pain, consider this your wake-up call. It's time to stop, for your health *and* for your back.

But not to digress. OK, now the weekend is over. You've spent it in plenty of company, by the way, since millions of people around the world are going to have back pain sometime this year. But millions of people will not have your advantages as you head off to your doctor's appointment: a clear mind, and this book in your hand. You have a mission—finding out explicitly what's wrong with you—and you won't just nod and go home if it's "nothing at all to worry about, probably just a touch of sciatica." You are going to decide on a treatment plan with your doctor that's as specific as the diagnosis you've received, since only after the pain is gone can you start the Backs in Motion program and begin working to prevent it from happening again.

Obviously the first step must be a diagnosis from a well-trained physician. If three days of rest, ice, anti-inflammatories, and some gentle movement like walking slowly around the block are already making you feel better, chances are your stiffness and pain will improve a little every day and you could be out of this in just a couple of weeks. But if it turns out to be something more serious, a disk problem or a stenosis that has finally erupted into pain, for example, you may need several months of physical therapy.

If You Need Therapy,
Do Your Homework First

Let your physician suggest some physical therapists, but don't just pick one off a recommended list. Meet with each one or, at the very least, make sure you know in advance what sort of practice the therapist has. If you're an active person, you want a therapist who works well with athletes and other active people. The way to find that out is to simply drop in and get a good look at the patients. If you see a roomful of men and women mastering the use of their walkers after hip replacement surgery, chances are you won't fit in very well. More important, your care won't be as aggressive as you might want. On the other hand, if you walk into a rehab center full of athletes building themselves up after knee surgery so they can get back out onto the field, that's probably the place you want to be.

Or take this shortcut: call the local professional teams and find out where they send their athletes for rehabilitation. Chances are they're using a strong physical therapist who understands what it means to be cut off from an active lifestyle and knows what it will take to get you back into yours.

Physical therapy can be as individualized as the injury, so it's hard to give you a perfect preview of what you'll be doing before we begin working together in part II of this book. But in general, expect mild exercises or a heat pack to help warm up cold muscles and get them supple, some stretching, and some "active" exercises to actually strengthen your back muscles. If it's the kind of injury that needs all the encouragement it can get to mend, your therapist might call up some technological troops or "modalities" like electrogalvanic stimulation—the "electric eels" of Hippocrates (remember?)—to increase circulation and speed healing. You'll also get a program to follow at home, and some kind of "back school" to teach you ways to lift and to move that are easiest on your spine.

This should get you well on the road to recovery. And this book will be waiting for you at the end. For it's only when you are essentially pain-free that you can start your personalized program in part II.

Maybe Massage?
Can Your Pain Be Rubbed Away?

Perhaps you got off light. The good news from your doctor is that you've pulled a muscle or ligament in your back and are beginning to get better already. For you, physical therapy might be like swatting a mosquito with a hammer, a much more overbearing program than you may need. Instead you'll probably start on your own exercise plan at home. But if you're still bothered by tense muscles that are spasming or are peppered with the painful trigger points, where muscle and nerve just keep antagonizing each other, a good massage therapist may be just what the doctor will order, especially if you're still able to play a sport while you're recovering.

At the Metropolitan Athletics Congress we see track and field athletes on the sidelines before and after events to provide whatever medical attention they might need. Massage is a common treatment for muscles that would otherwise be too sore to compete or that have come back from the contest tight and tense.

If your doctor has suggested massage as part of your back therapy, and you plan to have one or two sessions to get you through a race or match, remember the rules about sports massage. First, don't let anyone put oil on your body before an event, because it can prevent perspiration, a vital function for cooling the body. The pre-event massage should be short and should include lots of stretching so you don't get too limp and relaxed before toeing the line.

Afterward, the deep relaxation a thorough treatment can provide is an effective way to get some of the waste products of exercise out of your muscles and into your bloodstream, where they can no longer make you sore, not to mention relieving any muscle spasms. For the recovering back patient who doesn't happen to be an athlete, at least at the moment, the benefits of massage are pretty much the same: relieving trigger points and calming spasming muscles in the back, as well as increasing blood flow to the area to speed healing. But a massage twice a week is all you need. More than twice may bruise the muscles.

Massage is *not* anything-goes-as-long-as-it's-friction. Don't just go to someone who's willing to rub your body; do find a good massage therapist, which admittedly is not easy in many parts of the country. At the very least, make sure yours is a member of the AMTA—the American Massage Therapists Association—the national certifying organization. A state license to practice is a good sign, and it couldn't hurt to ask for the names of a couple of their clients for you to talk to.

Chiropractors? In This Book? Yes!

Hard to believe, I know, that an M.D. would voluntarily mention—never mind with a smile on his face!—the uses of chiropractic. The uneasy relationship between the two professions is legendary, but in fairness I must tell you this simple truth: just as there are good M.D.'s, there are good chiropractors. And they have, after all, been trained specifically in the structure of the back.

Nonetheless, even though some of my best friends are . . . I still don't believe the chiropractor's office should be your first stop in back therapy. Your M.D. should be your primary-care physician, your chiropractor should be your doctor's consultant. Go to an M.D. first and get a diagnosis. If your problem is one that responds to spinal manipulation—and there are such problems—and if your

M.D. is open-minded and understands how chiropractic can complement your medical therapy, you'll have the best of both worlds.

I wasn't always a believer, by the way. The change for me came when I was a fresh-faced physician not long out of residency and eagerly helping out at track and field meets in the New York area. It was there that I learned that chiropractors were practically indispensable. And when I discovered why, it was a little embarrassing to me. Apparently M.D.'s at the time were not much interested in turning out to help, so chiropractors were doing almost all the work. Small wonder they developed a following—deservedly so—and some track and field athletes swear by their chiropractors even today.

Still, my respect for chiropractic remained academic until one day during my fellowship training in sports medicine, when as it happens I had jumped quickly into my low-slung sports car in New York, late for an appointment in New Jersey, and sped off. Just seconds after cutting into fast-moving traffic, I looked in my dinky rearview mirror and saw a taxi rocketing up behind me, closing in for the kill. Naturally, I whipped my head and trunk around for a better look at what I was sure would be my last glimpse of the world. Zap! Suddenly I felt a sharp pain in my right lower back.

The taxi, of course, missed me by miles. But I was due at the New York Giants' team physician's office in just minutes, and there was a full day of patients ahead. As in Carly Simon's song, I didn't have time for the pain. So I continued to stop and start in traffic in the slow lane all the way across the George Washington Bridge and into New Jersey, knowing of course I was within minutes of passing the office of my friend Dr. Kenneth Ermann, the team chiropractor for the Giants. By the time I pulled up in front, I could hardly walk.

"Ken, you have to fix me *now*," I fairly whimpered.

Well, presto! With one quick adjustment I was on my feet and out the door totally free of pain. Apparently I'd had a facet joint that locked as I made that quick turn, and with one skilled chiropractic manipulation I was ready to go for the day.

It's a story I don't mind repeating, because there are many similar out-of-place problems besides facet syndrome (which responds better to chiropractic than to anything else) that chiropractors are qualified to fix. So if your doctor suggests chiropractic manipulation as an effective way to treat your back pain, don't be skeptical.

That is, of course, unless your new chiropractor breaks the news to you that you need to come back three times a week for the rest of your life. As my friends who are in the profession themselves say of such possessive practitioners, "Get out of that office quicker than you can say 'I need another sports chiropractor fast!'" Now and again, a case will realistically take a couple of weeks of treatment, but I don't believe in a lifelong program of manipulating spinal malalignment. Most good chiropractors don't either. They'll tell you to be prepared to come in once in awhile when something goes off, and that's all.

But what if your doctor recommends seeing a chiropractor and then leaves it to you to pick a good one? Again, you can often strike pay dirt just by calling the local professional sports teams to see whom they see. Considering what most of those athletes command for salaries, team management could hardly sleep nights letting them go to less than the best of anything—chiropractors included. Another way would be to call the American Chiropractors Association's Council on Sports Injuries and Physical Fitness at 1-800-593-3222. They can provide you with the name of someone in your area who has passed the American Chiropractic Board of Sports Physicians postgraduate boards in sports chiropractic.

Surgery: Not What It Used to Be

Surgery is the dreaded "S" word, the one that always scares patients when they hear it. It keeps people limping around for weeks or months instead of finding out what's really going on. They may not know much about back pain, but they do know this: no operation. "A neighbor's neighbor had one last year, or maybe it was the year before, and she couldn't get out of bed for two months. Or maybe she couldn't cut the lawn for two summers. I can't remember. Anyway, I'm not having any of *that*."

Well, think again. Certainly some types of surgery are more complicated and uncertain than others, but techniques have advanced tremendously over the years and

many of the once-complicated procedures are now relatively minor.

Surgery, sports doctors like to say, is the failure of all other treatment options. So we need a very sound reason for even considering it. What would my reasons be in cases of back trouble? I'd recommend discussing surgery with your doctor if you have "intractable" pain, that is, pain that just won't go away no matter what you've tried. Or if you've had any change in your strength or your neurological functions. In those cases surgical repair may be not only desirable, but necessary.

Fortunately, many procedures have improved by quantum leaps over just the last ten years. Now we have microdiscectomies for the repair of a herniated disk, done with the tiniest possible incision. You go into the hospital one day and go home the next. Within perhaps a few months you can be back on the playing field. The operation is brief, the tools used are bitty things, and the convalescence doesn't drag on forever.

Medical science now also has arthroscopic procedures done with minuscule scopes. And there have been many other surgical advances that can get you moving a lot faster than you might think. In skilled hands, the uncertainties just keep going down. In some procedures, back surgeons are now saying, the risks are so close to zero they can hardly be measured.

The best way to discover what might happen and what is involved is simply to ask the surgeon. No skilled doctor wants to subject a patient to an operation he or she

doesn't fully understand. Forthright questions get forthright answers. What are my risks? How fast will I be back to play? Will I be back to play at all? How many other active people like me have you treated? If you're met with astonishment instead of an answer—"Surely you don't intend to take up running again after we fix you up!"—find another doctor, one who understands you as an active person. And remember, if surgery is necessary, think of it as a beginning, not the end.

Are "Alternative" Therapies Real Alternatives?

What about all those alternative physical therapies and medical techniques you may have read about, or even had recommended to you by a well-meaning friend, who knows someone who got relief? Procedures like acupuncture, hypnosis, biofeedback, homeopathy, herbal medicine, Chinese medicine, yoga, and the so-called Alexander technique. Obviously I put my confidence in proven medical science, and I hope you will too. If your curiosity gets the better of you, I have no objection to trying them *in addition to* following your doctor's orders. But be careful of the "physical" ones that stress your muscles and bones. Yoga, a movement- and stretch-oriented therapy, can actually be harmful to people with spinal stenosis and some other conditions. Above all, let your doctor be your guide before getting involved. The other techniques just mentioned are muscularly and skeletally benign, so even though there's been no strong medical evidence proving their usefulness, I don't see how they

could hurt. If it makes you feel better to try them, go right ahead.

Sex: Playing the Indoor Sport, with a Bad Back

I see the question in my patients' eyes all the time. Some ask outright. Others don't. Most people I see are actually less afraid of having surgery than of not having sex. That's another groundless fear. Sex is just like any other sport when you're nursing back pain: probably no harm in playing, but you have to take precautions. Here's what this doctor orders.

In the acute stage, when the fear of pain is more powerful than the promise of pleasure anyway, it's true that you should skip the sexual acrobatics. But nobody ever said you had to be a gymnast to enjoy your partner. Lying on your back with a pillow under your knees and head and a rolled-up towel in the small of your back (see figure 3.1), you're ready for your partner to give you a thorough massage (this is not the time to fret about a massage license).

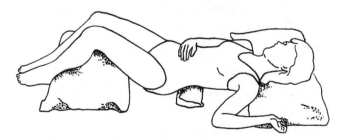

Figure 3.1

Thoroughly satisfying? I thought so. If you'd rather be on your stomach for your rubdown, put a pillow between your legs with your knees bent slightly to one side so that you're almost in a swimmer's sidestroke position.

As you start to feel better, experiment with some positions for intercourse that are easy on your lower back. Figure 3.2 is a good one for a woman who is comfortable in the pelvic-tilt position. She can support her back and hips with pillows to make this position more comfortable. However, it's not great for a man with back trouble, since the sitting position with pelvic movement puts too much stress on the lower spine.

The position in figure 3.3 is kind to the man's back, since he's able to keep it in a neutral, relaxed position. Women with back or neck trouble should avoid it, because both back and neck are twisted.

If back pain has become a family affair, figure 3.4 shows a posture that's good for the backs of both partners, so

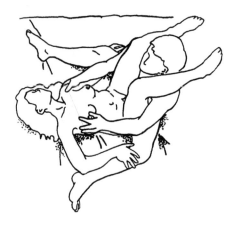

Figure 3.2

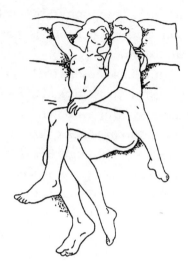

Figure 3.3

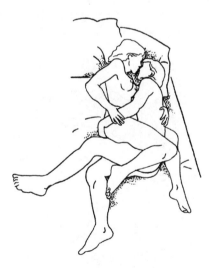

Figure 3.4

long as each one's neck is supported by a rolled-up towel or something similar. This position is not good for a woman with sacroiliac strain.

If the man in figure 3.5 keeps his back in a neutral position and uses his legs for thrust instead of his pelvis, he can be relatively pain-free. Unfortunately, it's nothing but trouble for a woman who has back pain.

The positions shown in both figures 3.6 and 3.7 are fine for either partner with back pain (except, again, for a woman with sacroiliac strain). The man, on the bottom, can support his lower back with pillows or a rolled-up towel and, for good measure, slip a pillow or two under his knees. Just right for the take-charge kind of woman, since the more work she does, the more he can baby his back. Besides, her position automatically puts her neck and back in a neutral position.

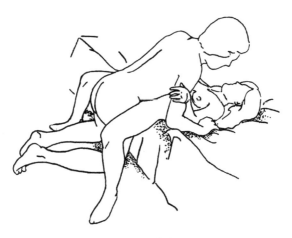

Figure 3.5

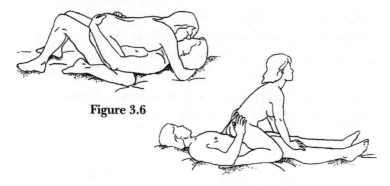

Figure 3.6

Figure 3.7

And finally, if you're not too exhausted already, there's the possibility shown in figure 3.8, helpful for the woman whose back is in a neutral or only slightly extended position. Skip it, guys, if it's your back that's bad. The back is too flexed for you.

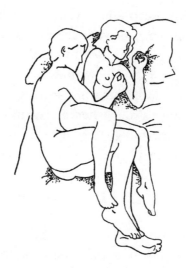

Figure 3.8

Somehow I don't think I have to worry about your completing the indoor sports part of your back therapy homework. I just want to drive home the fact that while you may have plenty to endure during your back pain convalescence, with a caring and understanding partner, a dormant sex life should not be one of them.

Aerobics and Nutrition: Can They Help?

Yes, they can. Even while you're recovering from your back pain—no, *especially* when you're recovering from back pain—you've got to eat sensibly and keep up your cardiovascular fitness. Remember that walk around the block about thirty-six hours after the discomfort first comes on? It's partly to help boost your conditioning. Be an aerobic pest of a patient. Keep asking your doctor what you can do during every stage of your therapy to keep your fitness from slipping as you focus on building up the pain-relieving back muscles. Upper-body ergometers in gyms can give you a great workout while sparing your spine completely. Swimming, as you've heard over and over, takes all weight off the back and gives your heart and lungs a fine run for their money. And yes, even nonimpact walks around the block will help preserve your aerobic conditioning so that when you go back to your sport, you're ready for it.

Nutrition is also important, especially when you're recovering. Even if you're temporarily on the injured list, keep up with your athlete's diet: low in fat, high in carbohydrate. Just trim your total intake if you must. Gaining weight inevitably puts more pressure on your back, and you certainly don't need that right now.

Let's Begin

OK. The worst is over. If you started this book with back trouble, you've taken my advice and done what you needed to do to get it under control. If on the other hand you're a "just in case" reader, you'll be an educated back patient should you ever need to become one.

Now we can get on with what you came here for: a personalized program for a healthy and pain-free back, based on the sports *you* play and how *you* move. In part II, I'll teach you how to design a back-care program for an active, athletic person, someone who makes regular demands on the body's machinery and in return is willing to give it the maintenance it needs to run well.

Someone like you.

Turn the page and let's begin.

The Backs in Motion Program

...*4*...

For a Healthy Spine,
Start at the Beginning

By now you're thinking of your back in a whole new way (or at least I hope so). This new perspective is as different from your old way of thinking as a black-and-white snapshot is from a color videotape.

Just as the videotape shows us a real, moving person, the Backs in Motion program illustrates that your spine is not a stiff model but an ingenious structure that expands, contracts, twists, and moves, separately and at times all together. Fittingly, the most important law affecting a real spine is Newton's law of motion. You'll probably remember it from high school science: a body in motion tends to stay in motion, and a body at rest tends to stay at rest, unless acted on by an outside force. Just substitute "back" for "body" and you'll begin to understand the constant demands you're making on your spine with the simple motion of getting up from a chair, for example.

But let me reiterate. Bones don't move bones. Muscles move bones. And Newton's law fights those muscles every step of the way, trying to keep stationary bones stationary and moving ones moving. Put another way, inertia is a very powerful force. Until you start thinking of your spine as being in constant motion (even as you breathe), it's a force that's easy to overlook completely, and that's how back problems get started.

Now, the "outside force" that makes your spine—and hence the rest of your body—move is your muscles. Muscles, attached to bones by tendons, stop and start every motion of your back, so they need to be fit and flexible enough not to get hurt while doing the job. At the same time, the ligaments between the bones need to remain tight for the joint to stay snugly aligned in order for the bones to move precisely in the smooth coupling that nature designed, not off-kilter, putting painful pressure in the wrong places. That's why the Backs in Motion program is specifically designed to increase muscle flexibility and strength. When you move—spiking a volleyball for all you're worth or simply taking a deep breath—the functional muscle-tendon-bone unit will move without creating stress on any of those individual components.

Since you've obviously come this far with me—through the relatively complex anatomy lessons and the sections on back discomfort—you'll be glad to know the rest is easy. The program, in fact, is as simple to follow as the equation below, which shows the four steps we'll be taking together toward a healthy back.

Basic 8 Foundation Exercises +
Your Individual Exercises + Aerobic Fitness +
Good Nutrition = A Healthy Back

Most back-care programs, or so it seems to me, rely on the same set of exercises. They more or less all condition the same muscles in the same way. This approach assumes that everyone moves in the same way, which is clearly not the case. And the strengtheners preparing our backs for the way we live are as individualized as we are.

However, just as every house, gracious colonial or sleek glass contemporary, has to start with a foundation, every back exercise program begins the same way. Those "foundation" exercises, which prepare the muscles we all use, I call the Basic 8. You'll find them in the next chapter. They will be familiar if you've already done a lot of reading about back problems. But now there will be a new twist. In my program the Basic 8 are just the beginning. For it's only with both the foundation exercises *and* your individual exercises that you can be protected in the most complete way.

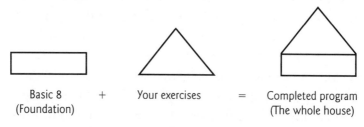

Basic 8   +   Your exercises   =   Completed program
(Foundation)   (The whole house)

Figure 4.1

The Basic 8 cannot be skipped. But without the individual exercises I offer, you will have no real structure. A hole in the ground with concrete walls and floor is not a home. Similarly, the Basic 8 are only the beginning.

Aerobic Fitness

But let us pause for a moment. Aerobic fitness matters too—a lot.

Now let me make sure I have this right, you might say. All I do is work on the correct muscles, and I'm safe from now on, is that right, Doc? Well, no, it's not. Just as you can't become a great soccer player by using nothing but a leg extension machine, you can't earn a healthy back simply by targeting a few muscles and getting them into shape. Leg strength is only part of the game of soccer, and muscle strength is only part of building a healthy back.

Remember our equation? If you're not aerobically fit, as well as strong, whatever good your newfound muscle strength from these exercises does, the reward won't last very long. In our Backs in Motion program the idea is not just to be healthy and free of pain. You should be fit enough to ride a bike or rake leaves without getting worn out right after you start. Fatigue, you see, is nature's way of saying your muscles can't keep doing what they're doing—at least not in the exact way they've been doing it. Keep going, nature is saying, and something's going to give. What gives first is your so-called biomechanics, your carefully groomed golf swing or tennis serve. You'll still strike the ball, but the muscles intended for the job are now tired and can no longer allow your body to maintain correct form. Other muscles are going to have to pitch in. Those backup muscles won't be ready, so they're likely to get hurt. And if those strained muscles have anything to do with your back, as they most certainly will, your back will hurt too.

Invest some time in your aerobic conditioning, and it will pay off. By training your body to burn oxygen effectively, aerobic fitness gives your muscles a reliable and steady supply of energy. Your muscles won't get tired as easily or quickly, so they won't give up as easily or quickly either. Fitness is an important part of both your life and your back wellness program, one that certainly deserves to be a part of your weekly activities.

Admittedly it hasn't always been easy to decide just what you have to do to be "fit." Originally it was thought that you had to dive into something major, like training for a marathon. Easygoing types disagreed, claiming that conscientious walking would do the trick. In 1990 the American College of Sports Medicine (ACSM), this country's Indianapolis-based central think tank for fitness research and recommendations, decided to give us the best and easiest-to-follow advice their researchers could offer. The ACSM published a paper explaining how much exercise is really enough, and what type is best for developing and maintaining overall fitness. The following guidelines were then quoted over and over, and they gradually became a kind of fitness bible.

If you wanted to maintain a healthy level of heart and lung fitness, a lean body, and strong muscles with plenty of endurance, the ACSM recommended a five-part program:

1. *How often?* The frequency of training should be three to five days per week.

2. *How hard?* Intensity should be between 60 and 90 percent of your maximum heart rate.

3. *How long?* Duration of training should be twenty to sixty minutes of continuous aerobic activity.

4. *What exercises work best?* Any activity that uses large muscle groups, can be maintained continuously and rhythmically, and is aerobic in nature. For example, bicycling, walking, running and jogging, skipping rope, rowing, stair climbing, swimming, skating, and various other types of endurance sports.

5. *Is aerobic training enough?* No. Strength training (resistance training) of a moderate intensity is also important to develop and maintain fat-free weight. The college recommended eight to twelve repetitions of eight to ten exercises that condition the major muscle groups, at least twice a week.

The ACSM point of view is very direct. If you wish to have more information, call the American College of Sports Medicine at (317) 637-9200 and ask for a brochure entitled *Achieving and Maintaining Physical Fitness.* In it you'll find step-by-step advice on starting and maintaining a fitness-oriented lifestyle.

Health Benefits Versus Fitness: The Difference

The more specific our fitness advice was, the more we recognized that some people just wanted to be healthy—and that the two were not necessarily the same. For instance, a fifty-three-year-old corporate executive who's lucky if he gets to walk down the hall to the next meeting and whose greatest worry is his doctor's stern warning about blood pressure and cholesterol doesn't require the same exercise program as his squash-playing colleague who does his own landscaping and takes the kids for bike rides every weekend. The goals are different, and we now know that in an exercise program, health benefits come a lot sooner and faster than fitness does.

Just a couple of years later, in 1993, it was time for more guidelines; you may have been among the many who wondered why the new ones seemed so different. The idea was not to confuse the new ACSM exercise recommendations with the five fitness rules mentioned above. The newer ones are easier for good reason. They are basic recommendations for general good health, not for robust fitness. Even the way these guidelines were announced makes that difference clear. The announcement was made in a joint news briefing with the Centers for Disease Control and Prevention and the President's Council on Physical Fitness and Sports, and the new recommendations were called a way to "fight America's epidemic of physical inactivity." In other words, these organizations wanted to get people healthier simply by getting them moving. The panel of experts recommended that "every American adult should accumulate 30 minutes or more of moderate-intensity physical activity over the course of most days of the week."

I couldn't agree more. Multiple research studies have proven again and again that those thirty minutes—which can be taken in bits as small as climbing a couple of flights of stairs, raking leaves, or walking at least partway to work—help ward off some frightening chronic illnesses, like coronary heart disease, high blood pressure, colon and breast cancer, osteoporosis, even depression. "The greatest health benefit is going from nothing to something," says epidemiologist Dr. Steven Blair, the ACSM's current president. And that was exactly who the recommendations were for: people who would be going from nothing to something.

Call it making a molehill out of a mountain for the sake of people who hadn't learned to climb yet. Dr. Russell Pate, a former ACSM president, explained the new approach succinctly when he said, "It may be that the current low rate of [exercise] participation is due in part to the public's perception that they must engage in vigorous, continuous exercise to reap health benefits. But actually the scientific evidence shows that even moderate physical activity can also provide substantial health benefits." While highly fit people probably enjoy some additional rewards, experts admit, the extra health returns diminish as fitness levels increase.

Well and good. While the Backs in Motion program won't have you sweating away like an Olympic hopeful, we do need to go beyond just tweaking your blood pressure and triglycerides. After all, this is a program for *active* people who want to be sure their backs are in the best possible shape for a day's activity that might include tennis, shopping at the supermarket, a workout at the gym, and finally home again to mow the lawn.

True, a dedicated channel surfer who wakes up one day and decides hereafter to take the stairs at work and pretend the elevator doesn't exist is going to earn some immense health benefits. But those benefits have little to do with muscle flexibility and strength. The channel surfer's oxygen delivery system will not be in a position to keep her muscles fresh and in good form for an entire eighteen holes, nine innings, or four quarters. Consequently, when you hear on the evening news that "experts say all you have to do to be fit is rake the leaves!" don't be misled. Yard work may increase your odds of good health, but if you want to enjoy that health with a problem-free back, you need to be *fit* as well, and there are no shortcuts.

Nutrition: Your Back Knows What You Eat

The French—who certainly have as much to say about the joys of good food as any people on earth—have a wonderfully wise saying that goes like this: "A moment in the mouth; an hour in the stomach; forever on the hips." I like to quote it to patients like Joanne, a thirty-four-year-old law student who came to me recently because of back trouble. Let me explain.

After a complete physical examination and workup, I could tell what Joanne's problem was. She was simply the most recent one in her family to suffer from an arthritic back, a prospect that terrified her, since she had already seen it put both of her retired parents into walkers. Too bad she wasn't terrified enough to do all she needed to do. For Joanne was one hundred pounds overweight, and although she regularly went to the physical therapy I prescribed for her back and claimed she did her at-home exercises to strengthen her muscles, she stuck to the same old diet—which is to say, no diet. Her weight, every extra pound of it, stayed on and overloaded a spine already predisposed to acting up. In truth, overweight as Joanne was, she couldn't really do much more than dabble at the exercise program anyway, and consequently her muscles never really became toned. Though I realize that developing good eating habits and practicing careful meal choices are probably somewhere below "write home" and "do laundry" on the lists of busy law students, Joanne knew that I might not be much help if she couldn't help herself.

So I called in my secret weapon, Heidi Skolnik, M.S., nutrition consultant to the New York Giants and New York Mets. Skolnik is not just vice president and director of nutrition for Plus One Fitness Clinics in New York, she is one of a gifted few who can make meeting precise nutritional goals seem as simple as adding a column of figures. Skolnik convinced Joanne that all she really had to do was keep a rough running total of carbohydrate grams during the day, and if she stayed within reasonable guidelines, the rest would take care of itself. Joanne did, her weight started coming down, and her back began rewarding her for the effort.

At a recent sports medicine conference, I talked about sports nutrition, which is nothing more than good, sound eating. Healthy eating means you're getting 60 to 70 percent of your diet as carbohydrate, 10 to 15 percent as protein, and 20 to 25 percent as fat. Sounds good, you say, but what does it look like on the breakfast, lunch, and dinner plates? If I have to write everything down and keep three running totals, I might as well invite my accountant to share all my meals! Right. Unless you turn into your own food cop, how *do* you decide during the day what to eat to get to those percentages?

Fortunately there's a simple and workable solution. First, translate what you're eating into carbohydrate grams, a fairly easy job, since it's printed right on the new food labels. Then, sharpen your pencil to figure out how many of those carbohydrate grams your body needs. First you must know approximately how many calories you eat daily. Then multiply that figure by 60 percent and divide this number by four, since four calories equal one gram of carbohydrate.

Done! The result is your daily carbohydrate need, in grams. See table 4.1, which gives you the number of carbohydrate grams for either a 60 percent or 70 percent diet, at various calorie levels. For example, two thousand calories a day multiplied by 60 percent equals twelve hundred calories. And twelve hundred divided by four equals three hundred grams of carbohydrate, just as the table says. Total up the carbohydrates from the labels of the

foods you eat each day, and if you come up with three
hundred, you've approximated 60 percent carbohydrate.
What about the other percentages? That's the nice part:
they usually fall in line closely enough all by themselves.
But fat still needs watching. Read the labels.

TABLE 4.1

Caloric Amount	60% Carbohydrate Grams	70% Carbohydrate Grams
1,500	225	263
2,000	300	350
2,500	375	438
3,000	450	525
3,500	525	613
4,000	600	700

For most people, those simple calculations work well.
But the more active you are, the more likely you may be to
know that since your body burns mostly carbohydrates
while you're exercising, two people of the same weight can
require widely differing amounts. The harder you work
out, and the heavier you are, the more carbohydrate
grams you need to keep muscles fueled.

And you can take all of this into account without ever
getting your calculator out of the drawer. Use table 4.2
instead. Look up your weight and find the number of carbohydrate grams you should be eating for your weight and

workout schedule. You don't have to convert a thing, even though the three columns are in the conventional metric units based on the number of carbohydrate grams you should eat per kilogram of weight. (If you're an ultra-precise person, you can extrapolate between the printed weight values to get a more precise carbohydrate gram total.) By the way, one kilogram equals 2.2 pounds, in case you want to double-check the table's math. For example, if you weigh 120 pounds, divide by 2.2 and get 54.5 kg. Multiply that by five and you'll get 273. By six, you'll get 327; and by eight, 436.

TABLE 4.2

Weight (Pounds)	5 Grams per kg	6 Grams per kg	8 Grams per kg
110	250	300	400
120	273	327	436
130	295	355	472
140	318	382	509
150	341	409	545
160	364	436	582
170	386	464	618
180	409	491	655
190	432	518	690

Keeping in mind how active you are, select the column that applies to you. If you exercise for about an hour a day, you'll need somewhere between five and six grams per kg a day. If you're out there for a couple of hours at a time, exercising hard, an eight grams per kg diet is probably closer to the mark.

Still a little confused and looking for a helping hand in planning your own day-to-day diet? Reach for the phone. The American Dietetic Association has a group of specialists who go under the name of SCAN (Sports and Cardiovascular Nutritionists), registered dieticians who are knowledgeable about sports nutrition and can help you. If you want to talk to a nutritionist in your area, or if you have a couple of questions about eating for your activity level, call the American Dietetic Association's hotline at 1-800-366-1655.

Ready, Set . . .

Our classroom work is finally over. No more lectures about what you should and shouldn't eat and how you should and shouldn't take care of yourself—though I hope by now you understand that as a sports medicine specialist, I could not just give you a couple of exercises, a pat on the back, and send you home. Active people need to understand how *everything* they do affects the health and strength of every part of their body—and especially the back.

So, let's put it all into practice. You're now ready to start on the program.

...5...

Laying the Foundation: The Basic 8

Even though the exact way your *back is put together* and the exact way *you* move it are unique and deserve a maintenance program to match, your spine still has a lot in common with everyone else's. Strong abdominal muscles, supple hip flexors, and firm butt muscles help make everyone's back flexible and sound. There are inescapable demands every one of us makes every day on the spine's "support system," demands that we can all prepare for in the same way.

And prepare we must. You can't just start nailing a house together on bare dirt without first laying the foundation, and you can't launch right into your custom back-conditioning program without first putting down a firm base of physical conditioning. No point building a steel-reinforced concrete fortress on some California hillside if the foundation is a flimsy, knock-together footing. One good, strong, Pacific rainstorm will send the whole thing on a muddy downward slide. In the same way, you can't just jump into your sport-specific back-training program without first shaping up the muscles that underpin the whole thing. You wouldn't spend week after week at the gym working on a powerful upper body, only to ignore the legs that support it, would you? Same thing applies here.

If you want your back to move easily, effectively, powerfully, and painlessly, step one is to target the basic muscle systems, the key "marionette strings" if you will, and get to work making them limber and strong. That's just what the Basic 8 exercises here will accomplish. Plan to do them at least three times a week, ten repetitions of each exercise, skipping at least one day between sessions. Think of them as the foundation for your individualized exercises.

A note about the drawings that go with the exercises that follow. I drew them myself because I wanted them to be just like those I draw in my office for my patients to help them remember the specific exercises and stretches I give to them.

The Basic 8 for Everyone

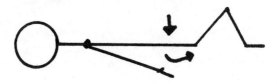

1. *Pelvic tilt*—stretches abdominals, stabilizes pelvis. Lie on back, knees bent, feet flat on floor, arms at your sides. Flatten small of back against floor (hips will tilt upward). Hold. Concentrate on doing most of the work with your abdominal muscles, not your buttock muscles.

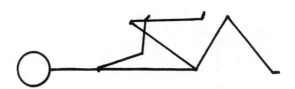

2. *Double knee to chest*—stretches hip, buttock, and lower-back muscles. Lie on your back, knees bent, feet flat on floor, arms at your sides. Raise both knees, one at a time, to your chest, and hold with your hands. Lower your legs to the floor, again one at a time, and rest briefly.

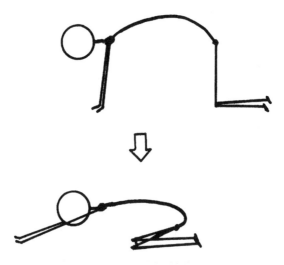

3. *Trunk flex*—stretches back, abdominal, and leg muscles. On your hands and knees, tuck in your chin and arch your back. Slowly sit back on your heels, letting shoulders drop toward floor. Hold.

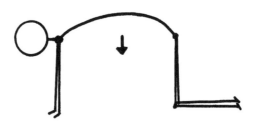

4. *The cat*—strengthens back and abdominal muscles. On your hands and knees, head parallel to floor, arch your back and then let it slowly sag toward floor. Try to keep your arms straight.

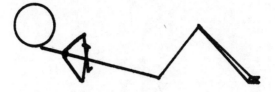

5. *Partial sit-up*—strengthens abdominal muscles. Lie on your back, knees bent, feet flat on floor, arms crossed over chest. Keeping your middle and lower back flat on the floor, raise your head and shoulders off the floor and hold. Gradually increase your time in the hold position.

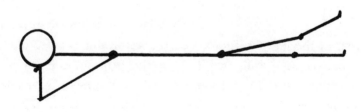

6. *Hip extension*—strengthens and stretches hip, buttock, and back muscles. Lie on your stomach, arms folded under chin. Slowly lift one leg—not too high—without bending it, keeping your pelvis flat on the floor. Slowly lower your leg, and repeat with other leg.

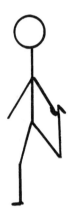

7. *Quadriceps stretch*—stretches large muscles of upper front of the leg. Standing on one leg like an ostrich, pull the other foot up behind you to your buttocks. Hold. Repeat with other leg and arm. If one-legged balance is tricky for you, do it this way instead: Lie flat on the floor on your stomach and pull your foot up as far as possible behind you. If you can't yet grab your foot, lasso it with a belt or towel, and then pull. Repeat on other side.

8. *Hamstring stretch*—stretches large muscles of upper rear of the leg. Sit sideways on a comfortable surface like a bed or low wall, one leg on the ground, the other stretched straight out before you and fully supported along the edge of the surface. Bend down slowly as far as you can comfortably go, and hold. Repeat on other side. If that's too high for your leg, then rest it on a low stool instead, and bend forward gently.

None of these "foundation" exercises is especially difficult, but you may find one or two of them a good deal harder to do than the others, at least at first. Believe it or

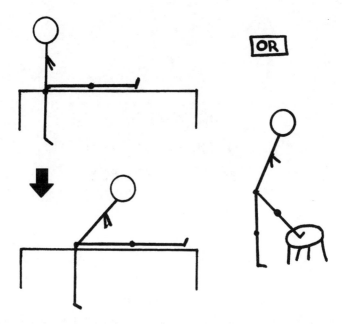

not, that's OK. If you could sail through all eight in perfect form without blinking an eye, I'd congratulate you on being one of the handful of people on this planet with either the youth or the genes to stay supple and strong by just walking around. If you're one of those rare people, you can just put this book down and cross back trouble off your list of worries. But having to work on these exercises instead means you're a member of the great majority—people with tight muscles, or with one muscle in a pair stronger than the other, or with joints that haven't been taken through the range of motion they were designed for in years.

So start working on the Basic 8, a minimum of three times a week, and as you lay that foundation for a healthy back, let's also begin your personal program in chapter 6.

...*6*...

Be Prepared!
The Athlete's Sport-by-Sport
Back Exercise Guide

See if one of these descriptions sounds anything like you. Perhaps you're a golfer who couldn't break into a run even if you were chasing the last taxi in town. Or a runner whose bicycle hasn't been out of the garage for years. Or the parent of teens who goes where the kids go, from the ski slopes to the pool at the Y to the tennis courts at school, when you'd prefer a nice long, easy bike ride instead.

Good, because you're about to find just what your back needs to stay in shape, to be ready for the way *you* use it, for the way you want to live and want to move. It's time to tailor your custom program, to put your "house" on the foundation, as we said in chapter 4.

In the last chapter, the Basic 8 exercises gave you the footing for any back-conditioning program. They ready muscles we all use, all the time, for the most basic everyday activities, working especially on the muscles most likely to trigger back trouble in most of us. But of course you're not "most of us." So now it's time to home in on *your* back, and the specific way you, an active person, move it.

What follows here is a sport-by-sport series of exercises that will prepare that "straw and paper cup" of yours to be active, healthy, and pain-free. In chapter 1 of this book, you may remember, there is a new, more accurate way of looking at your back. Very basically, I said that your spine is like a straw running through the middle of a paper cup, and the cup is the muscles, tendons, and ligaments that surround and protect the spine, diverting stresses from it. In a sense, each sport requires slightly different conditioning for the cup. But even if you're the kind of omnivorous athlete who has to try everything in the sporting goods store, from skis to skateboards, there's a good deal of overlap among sports where your back is concerned, as you will see.

Before we get started, let's also be clear about what this program *is* and is *not.* Will it make you a better athlete? Yes. A stronger athlete? Yes. A more injury-resistant athlete? By all means. It will do all of this by keeping your muscles toned and stretched, and keeping you in play. But we're not out to build you up to run a faster 10K or to boost your individual-medley swimming performance. That's up to your coach. The goal here is to protect your back, to keep you out there where you want to be, not home with a heating pad wrapped around your middle. Living actively and pain-free is what this book is all about.

But let's not get carried away. Follow the advice I offered Stephen, a forty-five-year-old attorney with a history of lower-back pain who breezed into my office just before leaving on an extended and much-delayed vacation. "I've been waiting a long time for this," he grinned and fairly salivated, "and I'm signing up for every sport that spa has to offer." Then he turned serious for a moment. "So, does that mean I have to do every exercise in your program?"

No. The point is to prepare your back for stress, and a half hour in a kayak, for example, hardly justifies weeks of getting ready for it. Stephen was not a professional athletc with the luxury of enough time to prepare for every little mishap. He needed to make some decisions. And so I simply said, "Use your judgment. Prepare your back for a sport to the same degree you plan on playing it. And that goes double if you're taking a serious plunge into something new."

Let's say you run every day to keep fit but have booked a fast-track week at a golf school to give your business career the boost you've promised yourself. In that case, you need to get busy. Start four to six weeks beforehand with the golf exercises before you step up to that tee. Surprising your back with a major new stress can only lead to a strain. So be prepared, and be ready.

Many sports, of course, use similar back movements, and therefore I have grouped these together, with exceptions mentioned in the exercise advice. However, please remember, no matter what your sport or sports, no matter how active or inactive you are, *everyone* does the Basic 8 at least three times a week. Then you add to the Basic 8 your individualized routine from the following action plan.

All of the exercises are illustrated and explained, with detailed instructions at the end of the chapter.

Let's get going.

Running/Jogging/Sprinting/Walking/Hiking

The Program: Exercises 1, 2, 3, 4, 10A, 10B

I group all of these sports together because in each one you're on your feet, you're moving forward, and many of the demands made on your spine are the same.

But not all. Obviously running, jogging, and sprinting are more stressful on your back than are walking or hiking. The jarring and impact they produce are not always well tolerated by spines susceptible to back pain, compared to walking, which is relatively gentle. So running, jogging, and sprinting require a couple of extra exercises, as you'll see.

Keep in mind that the most common cause of back pain in runners is not a vulnerable spine at all but a leg-length discrepancy causing low-back muscular strain. Take a longer leg and a shorter leg out for a run, and you can imagine the side-to-side tug-of-war going on at your hip and back muscles. No back exercises can fully steel you for that. So if you feel back pain coming on, first see your sports medicine doctor to determine if perhaps it might be starting in your legs, not in your back. If it is, you're fortunate. This condition can be easily corrected with orthotic devices that slip into your shoes, or perhaps with just a heel lift.

In the Basic 8, you've already done pelvic stabilization exercises and good stretches of your hamstrings and quadriceps. Runners, joggers, and sprinters need to add strengthening of the quadriceps and of the hamstrings that power so much of their movement. Your hamstrings must be strong enough for the job so that other muscles don't have to strain to help out. Exercises 1 and 2 achieve this. Three times each week do five sets of ten repetitions, with a weight that will let you just get to repetition five or six in the fifth set before you can do no more. And don't undo all your good work afterward with flimsy or worn-out footwear that sends the pounding of the road right up your legs and into your back. Let your sports medicine specialist or podiatrist recommend a good running shoe with lots of cushioning for protection.

Your calves and Achilles tendons may seem miles away from your back, but if they're not nice and flexible, along with the iliotibial band (ITB), which runs along the outside of your leg from the hip to below the knee, the tightness can actually stress the muscles of the lower back. So add the ITB stretch (exercise 3—more about this below) to your routine, plus the wall push-ups (10A and 10B).

If you're prepared for running, jogging, and sprinting, you're certainly ready for walking, which sends far less impact to the back. But do prepare for it. I wish I had a dollar for every patient who launched a walking fitness program convinced that the only possible risk in such a benign exercise might be slipping on ice. Walking works your back, as well as the rest of you. It deserves preparation.

In particular, walkers tend to get ITB friction syndrome. The ITB is a band of connective tissue that runs from the pelvis downward along the outside of your leg. Its basic job is to hold that limb from going too far out whenever you push your hip to the side, but if it gets tight, it can rub against either a bone in the hip or one down at the knee.

After awhile you get what doctors call a "friction syndrome" and patients call "one really sharp pain." So sharp you're tempted to soothe it by leaning or listing to that side, throwing your back off balance and triggering—what else?—back discomfort. Even the stabbing ITB pain may itself seem to cause back trouble as it radiates from the hip outward. The simple ITB stretch in exercise 3 can help prevent that.

Hikers can also prep with exercises 1, 2, and 3 to get their "propulsion machinery" toned, but hikers often put an extra load on their spines when they carry backpacks. Get ready for that load with a good back extension program at your gym, using a machine of the same name (exercise 4). Or mimic the exercise at home, holding a couple of heavy books to your chest like bags full of groceries, sitting forward on a stool, and duplicating the machine's straightening-up motion. Do five sets of ten repetitions, using a weight that will let you just get to repetition five or six in the last set and no further. If you cruise right up to ten on the fifth set, you're taking it too easy and need to add a plate on the machine (or find some heavier books at home). If you can struggle only to rep one or two, you're overloaded and should decrease the weight.

Swimming

The Program: Exercises 1, 2, 4, 5, 6, 7, 8

If swimming is practically a back-care program all by itself, since floating in water protects the spine, taking the weight and stress off the back, why do you have to prepare for it?

Not everyone does. Most of my patients who swim don't need any preparation beyond the Basic 8. But there are always the ones who say, "Doc, one of the reasons I'm in the water to begin with is that I want absolutely nothing to do with a bad back. I've been through that once before, so I know I'm always going to be a candidate, and whatever it takes to avoid trouble from now on, I'll do it. Any suggestions?"

Yes. Even though most indoor pools are relatively warm, your muscles still start out cold. And if you're on a regular swimming program, your workout yardage is probably significant—certainly significant enough that you wouldn't want to regularly push unprepared muscles into doing it. So warm up and stretch first. At the Downtown Athletic Club, where I'm Chairman of Sports Medicine, we've put stationary bicycles right alongside the pool. Smart swimmers use them for about fifteen minutes to work up a sweat and increase their body temperature by that all-important half a degree that helps steel-stiff muscles turn into nice warm, pliable taffy.

Next they do the Basic 8, plus what I call the judo pull (exercise 5), since I learned it in judo class back when I was six years old. The judo pull helps strengthen scapula muscles and stretch out shoulder muscles. It's simple. Just put your arms straight out in front of you, then pull them back to both sides in a quick, jerky motion, keeping your hands facing forward and forearms parallel to the ground. Fast now—six in a row in about three seconds.

Don't stop there. Considering what a weak scapula can do to a swimmer's back, it's worth doing some extra work to beef it up and stretch it out. Physical therapist Claudia Koziol is one of the most accomplished I've ever met, and in her opinion swimmers can't do better than exercise 7, originally developed by Shirley Sahrmann, Ph.D., P.T. (so around my office, at least, it's "Shirley Sahrmann's Scapula-Strengthening Exercise as Taught to Me by Claudia Koziol." But "exercise 7" will do fine for our purposes). Simply stand with your back against a wall, arms in the "hands-up" position, upper arms parallel to the ground. Keeping a right angle at the elbow, slowly bring your hands together over your head, then back down, ten times.

Total body stretch, exercise 6, is also a wonderful exercise for swimmers. Lie down on the floor, or even in the water, floating on your back, point your toes down and your fingers up and *stretch* your arms and legs as far as you can in both directions, holding for twenty seconds. Do this four or five times to stretch out your thorax, upper chest, abdomen, legs, and arms, to get them all ready for the swimming motion.

Trunk rotation (exercise 8) is another good preparation for swimmers because it mimics the upper-body roll that propels the freestyle stroke. Simply take a broom handle or mop handle (unscrew it from the broom or mop first!), and put it over your shoulders. Place your hands over it and twist from side to side twenty times, slowly, as far as you can in each direction. Next, bend over thirty degrees and twist twenty times from side to side again.

Finally, swimmers can benefit from a regular program of back extensions (exercise number 4), developing the muscles that work especially hard in the butterfly stroke and in many of the kicking motions.

Sound like a lot for a sport that's supposed to be "back-safe"? Well, it is. And for swimmers, this program represents the ideal. If you're already working out in the pool free of back problems, rest assured that you're in a sport that uses all of your major muscle groups, and if you have time to do only one set of exercises, the Basic 8 will be enough. The rest are superprotective extras for the especially back-wary.

Cycling

The Program: Exercises 1, 2, 3, 4, 6, 8, 9, 10A, 10B

The first exercise I often recommend to cyclists with back pain is a ride to the bike shop. Because the single most frequent source of trouble in this sport is equipment that does not fit properly. A professional will customize everything from seat position to pedal type to handlebar stem length, but if that seems too ambitious for you, at least check your seat and handlebar height, since both will determine whether or not your back is in its optimum position.

Seat height is defined as the distance from the top of your saddle to the spindle of your pedal when the pedal is down and in line with the tube that supports the seat. There's a serviceable formula for calculating it: multiply your inseam by 1.09. If you don't want to get out your calculator and measuring tape, there's an even easier way. With your heels on the pedals, extend one leg until the crank is at the six o'clock position. If your leg is barely straight, your seat height is correct. If it's not, adjust your seat just one-quarter inch at a time, taking several rides before deciding to change it again.

Fore-and-aft adjustments can be made too, within a range of about an inch and one-half. Again, the rule is simple: with the pedals in the three o'clock and nine o'clock positions, a vertical line from your tibial tubercle (the bony bump just below your kneecap) should cut right through the axis of the forward pedal. You have some slack in this adjustment, with a more forward position favoring "spinning" or quick, consistent pedal rotation, while farther aft should be better for cyclists who like to work harder in high gears.

In your basic bike fit review, you should also check your handlebar height. What cyclist—especially at the beginning of the season—hasn't straightened up and dismounted after a long and satisfying ride, and wondered how those muscles along the spine could have stiffened into position like slowly setting concrete? Even straight handlebars, which allow a more upright posture, the kind most all-terrain or "mountain" bikes are fitted with, require the back to do a certain amount of unaccustomed flexing. Does this matter?

Well, to a lot of backs, it does. In one study I saw recently, almost two-thirds of the riders involved in long-distance cycle touring reported at least some discomfort. For more than 20 percent of these riders, the problems were significant. Assuming these were cases of cycling-related discomfort and not caused by something else, one of the things I might have prescribed would have been some "handlebar therapy."

Two handlebar adjustments are possible, and both affect your posture and consequently the load your back muscles are under. Handlebar height is adjusted just as seat height is. Handlebar reach—the distance from the center of the bar

to the front of the saddle behind it—can be changed by re-
placing the stem that holds the bar with a longer or shorter
one. If your elbows are locked when you're gripping the
bars, the bike is too long for you, either because the frame is
the wrong size or because the reach is too long. On the
other hand, if your elbows are flexed more than 90 degrees
and your spine is quite rounded, the reach is too short.

Again, the rules of thumb are simple. Reach should
equal the distance from your elbow to the tips of your fully
extended fingers; handlebars should always be seat height
or, especially for racing, lower. The idea is to be positioned
in such a way that your body's weight helps do the work of
making the machine go.

All other things being equal, by the way, the "down" or
racing position on bikes with drop handlebars actually
helps stretch the back and build flexibility. But just as you
can overstretch muscles before a workout, you can do the
same thing on a long bike ride.

My advice is simple: If you've had a history of low-back
pain, skip the drop handlebars for all but short rides—rides
under fifteen minutes. But if riding is the only activity troubling your back, there's no reason for you not to use drop
bars. Just raise them bit by bit until the problem subsides.

Now that we've done the fine tuning of adjusting the bike,
what exercises will prep your back for trouble-free rides?

The most important is actually right in the Basic 8: "the
cat." In addition, since you're probably bent over much of
the time, give all of those muscles a real chance to stretch
out by adding the total body stretch (exercise 6) and the
back extension (exercise 4). Exercise 8, trunk rotations

(both upright and bent forward), are also helpful for stretching out your upper body.

Given the frequency of neck pain in my cycling patients, it's a good idea to invest some time in upper-spine flexibility as well. Simple neck stretches may be all you need (exercise 9).

Finally, in cycling, as in so many sports, the origins of back pain are not always in the back. Stiff leg muscles have a way of tightening the spine too, so keep your legs both strong and flexible with the quadricep and hamstring exercises (exercises 1 and 2) and the ITB stretch (exercise 3). Wall push-ups 10A and 10B keep the calves and Achilles tendons nice and flexible to avoid cramping and pain that ultimately affects the rest of your riding posture.

Skiing

The Program: Exercises 1, 2, 3, 4, 8, 10A, 10B, 11, 12, 13

"I'm off to hit the moguls, Doc. See you later."

Alas, you'll probably see me a lot sooner than you may think. I'm sorry to have to tell you this, but if you insist on combining aggressive, high-impact skiing (i.e., moguls) with a temperamental back, no exercise will give you the protection you'll need. So unless you're prepared to ski in a suit of armor, I'd recommend taking a trouble-prone spine onto the cross-country ski trails instead, or at least limit yourself to the less-death-defying and better-groomed Alpine trails.

But if you have no trouble with back pain and the snow is falling (or the boat is waiting and the lake is warm—for waterskiing takes exactly the same preparation, as does snowboarding), have a ball. Your preventive program is the Basic 8, plus strengthening your legs with quadricep and hamstring strengthening exercises (exercises 1 and 2), a good stretch for your ITB (exercise 3), back extensions (exercise 4), and trunk rotations (exercise 8). Calf stretches (exercises 10A and 10B) also should be done.

Your quadriceps need to be at their best so that your back can relax during the partial crouch of skiing, which requires the muscles to be fit, for balance and control. For quad toning, my skiing patients all swear by the wall sit (exercise 11), where you pretend you have a chair against the wall but you don't. You sit kind of in midair, watching an episode of your favorite soap opera from beginning to end if you can manage it. Though this exercise looks easy, it's quite difficult. In the beginning you'll be lucky to be able to stay in position for more than a couple of seconds, and you'll feel the pull on the inside and outside of your knees, where the quadriceps are being strengthened.

Start slow with a couple of minutes a day, and work up to a half hour. It can be done.

The ski agility drill (exercise 12) will help tone the take-off and landing muscles that control your torso on those fast runs. Mark a line on the floor and leap sideways from one side to the other, as shown, twenty times. This will help build sideways agility as you shift your weight again and again from side to side, which is what you'll be doing as you swoop down the mountain.

If your ski trip just isn't a ski trip unless you *do* get on that mogul run, at least get busy on exercise 13, ski plyometrics.

Plyometrics are rapid-fire muscle-conditioning movements that mimic the precise way your muscles function in any given sport. For skiing, get a small, sturdy box and simply leap onto it and back down again about twenty times rapidly, with quick, snappy motions in both directions, up and down. Do it both facing the box and sideways to the box. Think *bursts* of motion. You jump onto the box from a fully flexed position, bursting out of it and up onto the box, then back down to a flexed position, then immediately up again.

And even though I just got through a stern reminder that I'm your doctor not your coach, I'll put on a coach's cap just this once and recommend the NordicTrack ski machine as a superb way of preparing yourself to ski in snow. It strengthens the right muscles and provides a good aerobic workout, as any coach will tell you, and it also works your arms and legs through a full range of motion, stretching as well as strengthening.

Tennis/Racquetball/Squash/Paddleball/ Handball/Ping-Pong

The Program: 1, 2, 3, 5, 6, 7, 8, 10A, 10B, 14, 15

Cutting left, leaning right, diving for the ball, fast backhands, stinging serves—racquet sports get your back in motion practically every way it *can* move. Your torso is your power center for all of it, so most especially in these sports you must be faithful about your Basic 8.

Next come the leg muscle strengtheners that tennis players need to do, for much the same reason runners do. Racquet sports keep you on your feet, your legs are in constant motion, and fresh, strong muscles stress the spine less than weak, worn-out ones. You'll want to build up your quadriceps and hamstrings and stretch your calves (exercises 1, 2, 10A, and 10B). A nice, loose ITB will protect you from painful friction syndrome, so you don't favor one side over the other (exercise 3). Judo pulls (exercise 5) will help get the shoulder ready for overhead motion, and trunk rotations (exercise 8) loosen up your torso-twisting muscles.

Still, a back-safe tennis game takes more than muscles that are strong and loose. It takes the agility to move them rapidly and safely. That's what the tennis agility drill teaches (exercise 14). Think of it as speeding up your nerves' ability to fire the tennis muscles quickly and strategically. My competitive type A patients actually love it, since they can clock their times around the hexagon and see who's fastest.

Another tennis exercise I recommend is even more tennis specific. Get a length of Theraband rubber exercise tubing from your local physical therapy center or surgical supply store. You'll find that it comes in yellow, red, green, blue, black, and gold, which is intended not to complement your decor but to designate the tubing's strength or resistance. Yellow is the easiest, gold the most difficult. Tie one end of a piece of Theraband to the strings of your tennis racquet, the other to a doorknob or anything else about that height that won't give way. Then practice your trunk rotation and tennis swing against the resistance. The special genius of this exercise is that it not only helps strengthen your back, it mimics your exact tennis movements, so the strengthening happens on the side that will do you the most good.

Aerobics/Step Aerobics/Stair Climbing

The Program: Exercises 1, 2, 3, 4, 6, 8, 10A, 10B

It's easy to see how aerobics, step aerobics, and stair climbing rose to the top of the fitness charts. You get all of your conditioning in a well-lighted gym where it never rains, freezes, or gets heatwave hot. Additionally, there's plenty of company and the exercises do the job for you. No wonder so many of my patients bent on losing weight do one, two, or all three.

Another reason is that all three activities are relatively easy on the back, as long as you avoid aerobics instructors who think your legs are really just nature's version of Detroit shock absorbers. High-impact aerobics, remember, is an appropriately named activity. And your back knows that even better than you do.

The simple Basic 8 will do most of the prep work to give general limberness and strength to the principal muscles. Just add quadricep and hamstring strengthening (exercises 1 and 2), plus trunk rotations (exercise 8), back extensions (exercise 4), as well as calf muscle stretching (exercises 10A and 10B)—especially if you're going to spend any time at all on that stair climber, which puts extra stress on your lower back and legs.

Wrestling

The Program: Exercises 1, 2, 6, 8, 16, 17

Wrestling is good business for back doctors, which is not necessarily good news for wrestlers. Not that you can't take precautions and prep the back muscles that are going to be thrown into action. You can. But since wrestling, alone among the sports we're covering here, is virtually continuous hand-to-hand combat—one-on-one pulling, twisting, bending, yanking—there is little a back doctor can do besides making sure all of your supporting back muscles are well toned.

Still, it's obvious that the stronger you are in your upper and lower extremities, the better prepared you'll be. So even though it's not my purpose to give you a full-body-strengthening program, which should come from your coach anyway, I can recommend the basic back protectors for mat men and women.

They start, of course, with the Basic 8, as well as trunk rotations (exercise 8) to stretch out the upper-trunk muscles. The total body stretch (exercise 6) will also help keep muscles supple and less susceptible to strain. You'll benefit from some hamstring and quadricep strengthening (exercises 1 and 2), and since the stronger your upper body the less you'll have to strain to get and keep the upper hand in your matches, you'll certainly need to do biceps and triceps curls (exercises 16 and 17).

Soccer/Football

The Soccer Program: Exercises 1, 2, 3, 4, 6, 8, 9, 10A, 10B, 11, 14

The Football Program: Exercises 1, 2, 3, 4, 5, 6, 7, 8, 9, 10A, 10B, 11, 14, 16, 17

I group these two together because of their below-the-belt similarities. Both are essentially running sports requiring plenty of agility and lower-extremity muscle conditioning. But since soccer players spend a lot more time charging up and down the field than they do in the huddles that can take up half a typical football game, almost all the soccer exercises I recommend are lower-body ones. The Basic 8, of course. Then add strengthening of both the quadriceps and the hamstrings (exercises 1 and 2), the ITB stretch (exercise 3), back extensions (exercise 4), trunk rotations (exercise 8), neck stretching (exercise 9), for heading the ball, calf stretching (exercises 10A and 10B), wall sits (exercise 11), which are also helpful for the knees, and the tennis agility drill (exercise 14), because you need fast-firing muscles just as much on the soccer field as on the tennis court.

Football is a tough sport for backs, not just because you can regularly land under a pile of heavy people or get run into head-on by a locomotive in shoulder pads, but because you are constantly using your whole body for strength and agility. Therefore back preparation is probably more vital for a football player than for virtually any other athlete. Professional teams, of course, have lavishly equipped weight rooms for beefing up the body head to toe, but for our back-specific purposes, the most important exercise to be added to the protection that comes from the Basic 8 is the back extension (exercise 4). Do that one religiously *at least* three times a week.

And don't expect to finish up on the back extension machine, throw on a T-shirt and shorts, and go play football with a nice safe feeling. You need to back up your conscientious back exercises with the conscientious wearing of good protective equipment. If you're playing seriously, make sure you're padding seriously too.

Basketball/Volleyball/Beach Volleyball

The Program: Exercises 1, 2, 3, 4, 5, 6, 7, 8, 9, 10A, 10B, 13

In basketball you're either jumping, steaming down the court—or out of the game. It's what we might call "lower-body intensive," much like soccer, and therefore it takes the same kind of lower-body preparation to protect your back from stress. But of course throwing yourself into that jump shot block in midair isn't exactly easy for your spine to ignore, so you've got to have strong and supple trunk muscles able to hold it in place. Put a gold star especially on the trunk rotation exercise (8), which is like a dress rehearsal for all of that rapid-fire twisting and turning your NBA-level ball-handling style demands.

The dozen exercises in this program will do all that, plus help hone your agility. The ski plyometric (exercise 13) becomes the basketball plyometric simply by adding the ball. Hold it in a flexed (crouching) position as though coiling to spring up and make a shot, then jump up onto the box with a quick burst, and back down the same way.

Attention, especially, volleyball players: do your total body stretches as though your back depended on it. Every time you reach for the sky and a quick, sharp spike of the ball, stretching your arm as far over your head as your body will allow, you'll be grateful for the preparation of this especially strong stretch.

Ice Hockey/Field Hockey/Lacrosse/ Rollerblading/Roller-Skating/Ice-Skating/Speed Skating

The Program: Exercises 1, 2, 3, 4, 5, 6, 7, 8, 9, 10A, 10B

For the most part, these sports require leg strength, spinal flexibility, and the ability to shift your weight aggressively from side to side repeatedly without your back minding it. Though the Basic 8 take care of basic back-protecting pelvic stabilization, you need to run through the program above regularly to keep leg drive, in a semicrouched position, from taking its toll on that elegant "S" curve known as your spine—which really does prefer to be erect.

Obviously you'll want toned and flexible quadriceps and hamstrings (exercises 1 and 2), and back extensions (exercise 4) will build strength not only for the down-low posture of most skatinglike sports but for the additional twisting and turning it takes to score with a hockey puck or lacrosse ball. The scapula-strengthening exercise (7) will also help.

Trunk rotations (exercise 8) are very important, for much the same reason, and you might even want to do those on one leg at a time to really pump up those twisting slap-shot muscles. (At least you don't have to go looking for a broom handle; your hockey or lacrosse stick will be perfect.) And for lacrosse players, there's another off-the-record trick that can help: attach your lacrosse stick to a doorknob as in exercise 15, tennis arm strengthening, and work on strengthening your arm movements.

Rowing/Canoeing/Kayaking

The Program: Exercises 4, 5, 6, 7, 8, 16, 17, 18

Most back-related troubles in these sports start with the shoulder. So on top of your Basic 8, you want to make absolutely certain that the shoulder is adequately stretched and strengthened so it can absorb stresses and not pass them along to the back. If you're in any way a paddler, you need to get busy on exercise 4 (back extensions), judo pulls (exercise 5) to help stretch out and strengthen the whole scapula area, as well as exercise 7, "Shirley Sahrmann's Scapula-Strengthening Exercise as Taught to Me by Claudia Koziol."

Total body stretches and trunk rotations (exercises 6 and 8) will also help your back provide the arm power and trunk rotation that safely move a paddle or an oar. Strong arms spare the back as well, so work in some biceps and triceps curls (exercises 16 and 17). But if you could do just one exercise on top of the Basic 8, it would have to be bent-over rows (exercise 18).

Weight Lifting/Bodybuilding/Home-Gym Exercise

The Program: Exercises 1, 2, 6, 8

"Whoa there, Doc. I'm already a weight lifter and now you're going to tell me what weights I should be lifting to protect my back?" Well no, I'm not. That would be a little like tutoring Mickey Mantle in the fine points of swinging a bat. Besides that, you might be surprised to hear that I've found weight lifters and bodybuilders to have few back problems if they faithfully lift with proper form. So for you iron-pumping types, just a reminder: don't get so wrapped up in strength that you neglect flexibility. Then you *will* have some back complaints. Stretch out your arms and legs (exercise 6); do the quadricep and hamstring exercises (1 and 2) after you work on your arms; do some trunk rotations (exercise 8) to stretch out your trunk muscles.

And oh yes: if you want to continue staying out of my office, wear your weight belt.

Golf

The Program: Exercises 1, 2, 3, 4, 6, 8, 10A, 10B, 19

The sport of running may fill up podiatrists' offices, but golf fills mine, perhaps because the connection to the back is more obvious in golf than in practically any other sport, or because people who already have back worries think they should take up this so-called easygoing game. I do know the most frequent question I hear is, "I have a [disk herniation, facet joint problem, on-and-off low-back trouble that feels like sciatica, or whatever]. Can I golf?"

Why not, if you're properly prepared? Since much of golf is walking—or should be, in my opinion—you need quadriceps and hamstring strengthening (exercises 1 and 2), and ITB and calf stretches (exercises 3, 10A, and 10B). But to make absolutely sure the back itself is ready, add on some back extension exercises (4), total body stretches (exercise 5), and trunk rotations (exercise 8) using your golf club—upright and at thirty degrees. When that's done, take the club from your shoulders and put it behind you across your waist, bend over to your customary address-the-ball angle, and do exercise 19.

Bowling

The Program: Exercises 1, 2, 3, 4, 5, 6, 7, 8, 9, 10A, 10B, 11, 16, 17, 18, 20

Yes, America's sport is back! Just check the parking lot at your local lanes some weekend. After languishing for years as a sport you thought you couldn't enjoy unless you owned at least one monogrammed satin jacket, bowling is once again family weekend fare and has even become an Olympic sport. So back problems cannot be far behind.

My advice: get at them before they get you. In addition to the upper-extremity strengthening of biceps and triceps curls (exercises 16 and 17) so you can hold the ball without straining your shoulder and, after that, your back, you're also going to do some stretching and strengthening of the scapula (exercise 7).

But bowling has one exercise all its own in my program—exercise 20, the bowling lunge—which shows you how important I believe it is to stretch the iliopsoas muscle of the inner hip. This lunge mimics your delivery of the ball down the lane, but you hold that position and stretch out the inner groin, opposite hand and leg, just like freeze-frame bowling.

Be careful about what size ball you pick up at the lanes if you don't own your own of the right weight. Don't be a hero and go for the heaviest ball you think you can handle, because you probably won't be able to—at least not without consequences to your back.

Track and Field

The Program: (Depends on you!)

Track and field athletes have one thing in common: they're all different. As medical director of the Metropolitan Athletics Congress and chairman of the Association Task Force on the National USA Track and Field Medical Committee, I see lots of track and field athletes performing. That's probably why so many adults, who've heard about the fine physical training and spirited peer competition track and field offers, come to me for advice.

But what do you say to the patient who walks in and declares, "I'm going to participate in my first track and field meet this weekend. What exercises should I do to protect my back?" I suppose you could do all of them, but then you'd have no time for your events. The real question is, are you throwing or running or jumping or pole vaulting or what? The best advice is what I gave attorney Stephen at the beginning of this chapter. Prepare for what you'll be doing, not for what you won't. Are you throwing the javelin and then going home? Are you just going to run the four hundred? Or the ten thousand meters?

I can't give you a better program than you can pick for yourself. If you're a thrower, go to the exercises at the end of this chapter and pick the ones that work your arms and upper body. If you're a runner, concentrate on the legs. Prepare, but know what you're preparing for.

And one more word to the wise. If you're coming in to see me on Tuesday for a meet this coming Saturday, and you figure why not sign up for two or three different events, you're too late. Either skip the meet or keep your fingers crossed. Next time give yourself about six weeks to get your back ready.

Martial Arts/Yoga

The Program: Exercises 1, 2, 3, 4, 5, 6, 7, 8, 9, 10A, 10B, 21

These Eastern disciplines work on the power of developing both flexibility and strength—which should sound familiar to you by now, since they're the exact qualities we're striving for in all of your back-related muscles. Even though the disciplines themselves are essentially a form of preparing your back for the stresses and strains of life, both martial arts and yoga practice can be pretty vigorous. So I don't recommend jumping right into them without a little preparation.

Do the Basic 8, certainly, for lower-extremity strength and flexibility, plus trunk rotations (exercise 8) to get you ready to do those quick and aggressive movements that are the staple of martial arts training. In fact, as you'll see from the extensive list for the martial arts and yoga program, even though I trust the safety of both martial arts and yoga for intermediates, I think they are too ambitious to just throw an unprepared back into. Work your way through this program first for two weeks, three times each week.

Sex (Yes! Sex Is a Sport Too)

The Program: Exercises 1, 2, 3, 4, 6, 8, 16, 17, 18

In chapter 3 I made you a promise that I need to partially take back. No, you don't need to be a circus gymnast to enjoy your partner, as I said—especially if one or both of you currently has back trouble. But now I want to qualify that remark. As long as you're both pain-free, it is in fact a good idea to be fit enough for some acrobatics.

No one knows for sure where passion will lead—at least not if we're lucky—and you may be on your way into some novel positions that will take both grace and strength to get back out of without aggravating your spine. Be ready for some spontaneity.

What's the best preparation? The Basic 8, of course, especially the pelvic tilts. Trunk rotation (exercise 8) is also surprisingly valuable, as are back extensions (exercise 4), the total body stretch (exercise 6), bent-over rows (exercise 18), which will help strengthen your shoulder, as well as biceps and triceps curls (exercises 16 and 17), for the kind of upper-body strength that will get you out of contortions that may have taken even you by surprise.

Time to Get to Work!

At this point you know just what needs to be done to give you a sports-ready spine. By now you may be thinking that twenty-one exercises aren't a lot, that maybe it would be simpler to just do them all and be ready for anything. I don't recommend it. You're going to be wasting time on work you don't need to be doing, and you'll have less time for the sport-specific conditioning your body also needs if you want to enjoy your cycling, running, golf game, or judo class.

Be specific. Do your Basic 8 for foundation work—very important—and add just the top your particular house needs. Then put the back stuff away and enjoy your tennis lesson or whatever. And if you're going on vacation, be specific about your sports agenda. Add in additional back prep exercises only for sports you'll be giving a serious try.

So you've got your plan. Now, as Nike says: "Just do it!"

Exercises

Do these three times a week, unless otherwise noted, at the same time as your Basic 8.

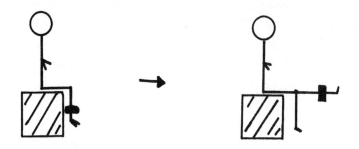

1. *Quadriceps strengthening.* Using the quadriceps machine at your gym, do one leg at a time (using both legs decreases the training your legs get). Five sets of ten, enough weight so you have to stop at rep five or six of the last set. (If you get to ten, you have too little weight. Add a plate. If you can't get past one, you have too much weight. Take a plate off.) Lift, hold three seconds, lower your leg slowly until the plate hits. Ten seconds rest between sets.

If you have problems with runner's knee, don't do the full leg extension. Instead start at the last thirty degrees (six inches) of the lift. That keeps the kneecap up out of the groove that it rides in, and protects you. Ask your trainer to show you how to set an extra pin in the back to "lock out" some of the machine's range so it gives you only six inches of terminal extension. (Or you can take a stool and build it up with books in front of you in your home gym so you have a place to stop.)

If you don't belong to a gym, sit up on a desk or other high surface. Take a gym bag or duffel filled with weights (books, soup cans, whatever) and strap it to the lower leg or hang it from the foot or ankle. Lift to full extension, hold for three seconds, then come slowly back down. Same sets and reps as on the machine, and same advice about weight. If you don't want to do full extension exercises, just use a stool as your stopping point.

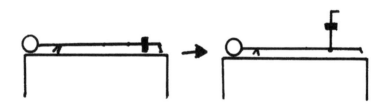

2. *Hamstring strengthening.* On the leg curl machine, again one leg at a time, five sets of ten with as much weight as it takes so on the fifth set of ten you fail (see exercise 1). Lift, bringing foot up to right angle, hold three seconds, slowly come back down. If you don't belong to a gym, just go to any good sporting goods store and buy a set of ankle weights that wrap around your leg with a Velcro attachment. Lie on a bed or on the floor, and duplicate the machine's motion.

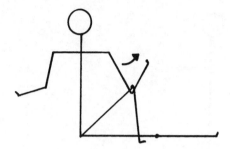

3. *ITB stretch.* Sitting on the floor, feet straight out, bring one knee up to your chin and place the foot of that leg on the floor just outside the opposite knee. Using the opposite elbow, push the raised knee across your body, hold for twenty seconds. Repeat with the other side.

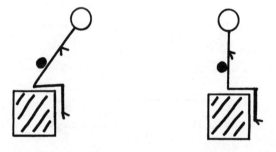

4. *Back extension.* Start in a flexed (bent) position on the back extension machine. Then push backward until you're straight up and down, a right angle at the hips. Hold for three seconds, then slowly come back down to the flexed position. Or mimic the exercise at home, holding a couple of heavy books to your chest like bags full of groceries, sitting forward on a stool, and duplicating the machine's straightening-up motion. See exercise 1 for sets, reps, weights, and rest.

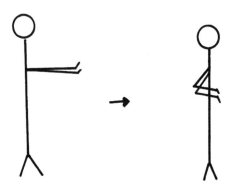

5. *Judo pull.* Start with your arms straight out in front of you, and in a quick burst of motion, pull them backward, bending your elbows, hands staying at shoulder height, then straighten them out in front of you again. Five sets of six, fast, every day.

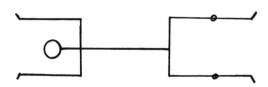

6. *Total body stretch.* Lie on your back, facing up. Stretch your feet and toes, and hands and fingers, as far as they can go away from you. You should feel the stretch all through your trunk and your stomach. You can also do this standing, reaching for the sky, up on your tiptoes, but it works best on your back. Five reps, hold for twenty seconds each.

7. *Scapula strengthening* ("Shirley Sahrmann's Scapula-Strengthening Exercise as Taught to Me by Claudia Koziol"). Standing with your back up against a wall, hands

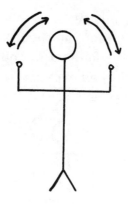

in the "hold-up" position shown, upper arms parallel to ground, slowly bring both hands up in a semicircular motion until they meet overhead (hold right angle at elbows), then slowly bring them back down so upper arms are once again parallel to floor. Four sets of ten, daily.

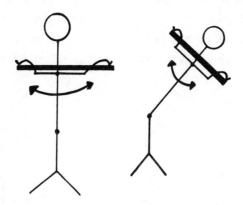

8. *Trunk rotation.* Take your broom handle (or hockey stick or golf club or lacrosse stick), put it over your shoulders, drape your hands over it as shown, and twist slowly as far as you can in one direction, keeping your pelvis straight ahead, then slowly to the other side. Hold for twenty seconds at the end of each rotation. Do five times, then bend thirty degrees at waist and repeat.

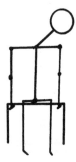

9. *Neck stretching.* Sitting in a chair, firmly grasp your seat bottom by your left hip with your left hand. First tilt your head toward the right (ear toward shoulder), then turn to look at your left shoulder, head still tilted. Pull up on the chair for about five seconds, relax for two seconds, then lean your body to the right for five seconds. Rest and repeat on the opposite side. Five repetitions each side.

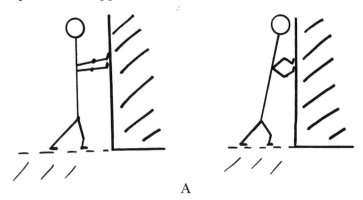

A

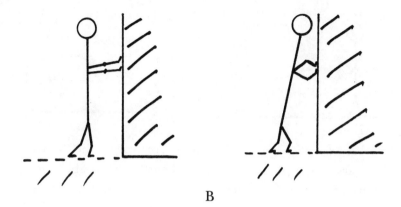

B

10A and 10B. *Wall push-ups.* Stand about two feet from a tree or wall, "good" foot forward, back straight, and foot you're working on behind you, heel to the ground. Lean forward into wall as though doing a standing-up push-up, hold for twenty seconds, and repeat ten times for each foot. Then repeat with the knee of the back foot slightly bent (10B), keeping the heel to the ground. You should feel that stretch lower down.

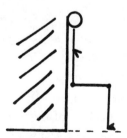

11. *Wall sit.* Simply sit up against the wall, knees at right angles. You'll feel the sides of the knees especially working hard. Hold for as long as you can. Try to get up to a half hour, maybe watching a favorite television show.

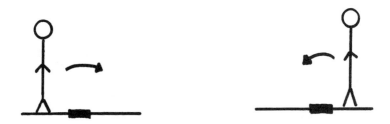

12. *Ski agility drill.* Putting a piece of tape on the floor as a marker, jump quickly back and forth over it about ten times. Start in a bent-knee position, then blast up into the air and land as far as you can on the other side.

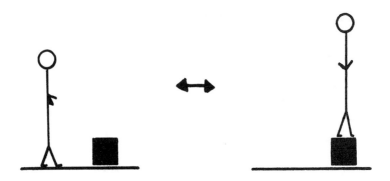

13. *Ski (and basketball) plyometric.* Get a small, sturdy box. Starting from a crouched position, leap up onto it, landing with knees slightly flexed, then come back down. Repeat with the box alongside, jumping both left and right onto it. Two sets of ten, in each of the three directions.

14. *Tennis agility drill.* Tape a hexagon onto the floor, about thirty-six inches per side. Starting in the center, feet together, leap to one, then leap back to center; leap to

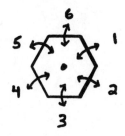

two, and back to the center; three, and back to the center, and so forth, until you've gone all the way around.

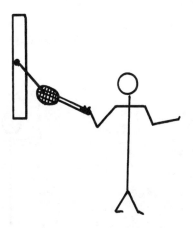

15. *Tennis arm strengthening.* Attach tennis racquet with Theraband tubing (see page 132) to a doorknob or other secure point about three to four feet off the floor. Hold the racquet as you normally would, and rotate your trunk just as if you were hitting a ball, until you meet firm resistance. Then hold for twenty seconds, and slowly reverse to your starting position. This can be repeated for backhand, if you want. Three sets of ten.

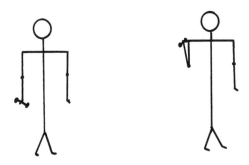

16. *Biceps curl.* Bend at the elbow, coming all the way up, holding for three seconds, then going back down to full extension. Do fifty reps per arm three times a week using a two-and-a-half- to three-pound dumbbell. If you can't manage that much weight at first, use a soup can.

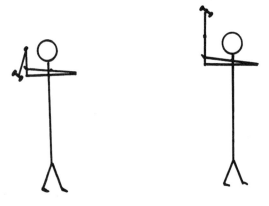

17. *Triceps curl.* Holding a two-and-one-half- to three-pound weight behind your head, elbow pointing upward and upper arm supported with your opposite hand, straighten arm, then bend again. Fifty reps, both arms. (You can use a soup can if you can't handle that much weight in the beginning.)

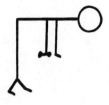 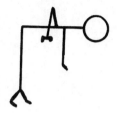

18. *Bent-over row.* Hold a three-and-a-half- to five-pound weight (working up eventually to ten or fifteen pounds), bent over at the waist as shown, torso parallel to floor. Bring weight straight up to shoulder height (elbow is pointing up), hold for three seconds, then slowly come back down. Fifty repetitions each arm.

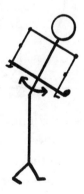

19. *Golf trunk rotation.* Holding a golf club behind you at waist level, bent over at the angle you'd use to address the ball, twist to either side, as in trunk rotation (exercise 8).

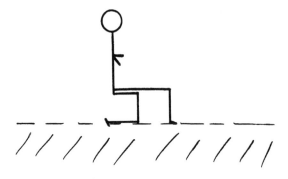

20. *Bowling lunge.* Drop down into bowling position, as shown; hold for a count of twenty, and stretch. Switch sides. Five reps each side.

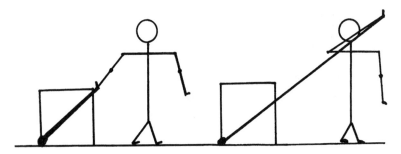

21. *Diagonal pull.* Attach a length of Theraband tubing (see exercise 15) to the bottom of a table or other secure point, then pull up in the diagonal motion shown until you can pull no farther, hold for twenty seconds, then slowly come back down. Twenty times, each arm.

...7...

Not an Athlete? Not a Problem: The Athlete's Back Program for Nonathletes

"*We're all athletes.* It's just that some of us are in training and some of us aren't." Absolutely true, though it took the late cardiologist and much-loved running writer Dr. George Sheehan to put it simply.

The human body was designed for motion, and move it we do. If your days consisted of nothing but shuffling from the bed to the TV room, to the dinner table and back to bed, you'd never have begun reading this book. Most of us have demands on our time. We buy groceries, do household chores, shop, iron, hammer nails, help a neighbor stack firewood, run for the bus—and as a result, in a sense, we're all athletes. And as an unofficial athlete, this back program applies just as much to you as it does to your neighbor who goes through four pairs of running shoes, or two sets of bicycle tires, a year.

Tennis pro or typist, one way or another, everything you do during the day makes demands on your back. Coaxing that wrinkle out of the rug in the hall, hanging on a sub-way or bus strap, pushing a shopping cart at the market, opening the hide-a-bed for visiting Aunt Sue—every single one of these motions uses muscles conditioned by the Basic 8. Therefore, you should be doing them as faithfully as any league-champion bowler. In a word, *sport* means motion, ways of moving and using your body not altogether different from what one would do all day long. So don't feel left out of a plan for a healthy back because you're having trouble thinking of yourself as an athlete. It's not your life you need to adjust, it's your thinking. Backs in Motion is your program too.

Read through chapter 6 again, especially the exercises at the end. This time look for all of the familiar movements you do all day without giving it a thought, and you will find the exact program *your* back needs. You just have to use your new way of thinking to equate exercise with ordinary movement. As I said in the last chapter, prepare for what *you* do, which means first understanding how virtually every detail of your daily living affects your spine.

Here are a few examples of common activities and the sports they resemble, but you can surely find many more in your own life. When you do, just turn to the chapter 6 exercises that cover similar motions, and add them to your program. And remember: *everyone* does the Basic 8.

Walking the Dog

Dogs may be loving, but they are not patient—try teaching forbearance to Snoopy the beagle on the scent of a squirrel. The leash snaps taut as piano wire, and your arm and shoulder go right along with it. Then suddenly, over there, his favorite terrier! And wow, she's in heat! Let's go! Yank, tug, a leap in the air.

Feeling like a lacrosse player in the middle of a tough match? You should.

None of this beagle energy hits your spine in a nice, predictable, straight-up-and-down way. Though the motions are mostly side to side, they're largely unpredictable. So the exercises that you need to do to be ready for them are the ones that prep you for walking (quadriceps and hamstring strengthening, exercises 1 and 2), as well as some back extensions (exercise 4), so that when Snoopy pulls, you can pull right back. Judo pulls (exercise 5) are important to help your shoulder be ready, while trunk rotations (exercise 8) will loosen your middle up for when it's time to twist, bend down, and clean up the telltale evidence of Snoopy's hearty dinner last night. And exercise 18, bent-over rows, will also work the dog-restraining muscles.

Prepare your back with exercises 1, 2, 4, 5, 8, and 18.

Reaching for Things at Home, the Office, the Supermarket . . .

One of my favorite "Far Side" cartoons shows a bewildered little child standing in the middle of a market where everything is way up on shelves near the ceiling, completely beyond reach. The place is called, of course, an *in*convenience store.

You probably go to a few of those yourself. Food shopping often takes the reach of an orangutan to get to the topmost shelf for a particular soup you want.

Back home again to wash windows, or later that week in an airplane you haul your garment bag out of the overhead locker—all of these movements are *reaching-type* movements, and they're not so very different from raising your arm to serve a tennis ball. To strengthen and ready your shoulders for home, office, travel, or shopping, do exercise 5, judo pulls, and exercise 7, the scapula-strengthening exercise, as well as the total body stretch (exercise 6), some trunk rotations (exercise 8), and neck stretching (exercise 9).

Not all reaching is up, of course, as anyone without a cleaning service can tell you. While scrubbing out the bathtub or stretching all the way under the sofa to retrieve Snoopy's ball, you're moving in a different way. If you're on your knees and reaching, for extended periods of time, the back extension exercise and the total body stretch (exercises 4 and 6) are especially good.

Prepare your back with exercises 4, 5, 6, 7, 8, and 9.

Pushing and Lifting

As far as your back and spine are concerned, the activity is not just vacuuming or running the snow blower or raking a few leaves. What you're doing is vigorous back-and-forth motions that derive most of their power from the lower back—even more so with motions such as shoveling snow or weeding the vegetable garden, taking out the trash, lifting junior out of his stroller, and grappling with the grocery bags. All are motions that should be prepared for.

And don't forget your legs—especially your hamstrings, quadriceps, and calf muscles—if you're going to be pushing a snow shovel, lawn mower, or grocery cart loaded with heavy canned goods. To prepare your lower back and arms for this sort of lifting, do back extensions and arm exercises.

Prepare your back with exercises 1, 2, 4, 5, 6, 7, 8, 16, 17, and 20.

Gardening

At one time or another, the gardener does it all: pushing, pulling, lifting, reaching—everything we've discussed so far. But there's more. Unless you have a secret weed-free process, or your seedlings jump into the ground all by themselves, you spend a lot of your gardening time on your knees, bent over. That's a lot like being on a road bicycle with drop handlebars, so the total body stretch (exercise 6) is as beneficial to you as it is to any cyclist. After crouching for as long as most gardeners do, you're going to feel an achiness in your back and you'll be surprised how good it feels to lie faceup on the floor and simply stretch that out.

Ah, but the day is probably not done yet. Time to put all three hundred feet of garden hose back onto that reel. Now *that's* an upper- and lower-back stressor, a little like the pulling and pushing of rowing, a little like the twisting and bending of golf. So prepare your back to do this work just as any rower or golfer would: back extensions, judo pulls, total body stretches, scapula-strengthening exercises, trunk rotations, and the golf trunk rotation bent at the waist (exercises 4, 5, 6, 7, 8, and 19). Bent-over rows (exercise 18) will also help.

And if that reel work, or whatever, is *really* uncomfortable, get yourself some Theraband (see page 132) and include exercise 21.

Prepare your back with exercises 4, 5, 6, 7, 8, 18, 19, and 21.

Painting the House, Waxing the Car

Up and down, wax and buff, did I miss that spot? Keep those arms moving until the car sparkles. Jobs like these are a lot like learning a martial art, which is exactly what Daniel, the Karate Kid, discovered in one of my son's favorite movies of the same name. Why just teach karate when you can double up and get chores done for you at the same time? Daniel's shrewd mentor calculated. So, "Wax on, wax off!" was one early lesson.

So was "Paint up, paint down!" It was karatelike motions being taught with a practical twist: the car just happened to shine and the fence looked much fresher after the first few lessons.

With all the balancing, pressing, reaching, bending over, and tilting sideways these jobs require, your vertebrae know they've done a good day's work. Make sure their "fitness survival kit" is ready. You need to prepare your shoulders for the occasional and regular sort of stress, and to limber up the trunk with trunk rotations (exercise 8).

Going up and down ladders is a lot like being on a stair-stepper, so you'll do some of the same lower-body exercises as the aerobic ones at the gym. In addition to your Basic 8, you'll add in the exercises below, including quadriceps and hamstring strengthening (exercises 1 and 2), the ITB stretch (exercise 3), and the calf work in exercises 10A and 10B. And because your neck can get achy and even spasm from too much of this kind of stress, add exercise 9.

Prepare your back with exercises 1, 2, 3, 4, 5, 6, 7, 8, 9, 10A, 10B, and 18.

Carrying Shopping Bags

Paper or plastic?" the grocery clerk usually asks.

It's more than a choice of ecological preferences. Carrying heavy loads up against your chest, as with chock-full paper grocery bags, is not the same as the suitcaselike position that handled shopping bags and plastic grocery bags allow. Both positions require low-back exercises—back extensions (exercise 4) as well as the full Basic 8—but holding bags high certainly takes more upper-body strength. The stronger your arms, thanks to biceps and triceps curls (exercises 16 and 17), the easier it will be to hold on. Strong shoulders will also help make the long, grocery-laden walk to the front door more comfortable, so in addition to scapular strengthening and stretching (exercise 7), plan on some bent-over rows (exercise 18).

Prepare your back with exercises 4, 5, 6, 7, 16, 17, and 18.

Doing the Laundry

Whoever said that washers and dryers should be on the floor? Certainly no back doctor. The constant bending and extending of your back as you load and unload those little caverns of cleanliness—up and down and up and down— are a lot like back extension exercises (exercise 4), but without the benefits you get on a back extension machine. More is going on. There's trunk rotation (exercise 8) while your back is flexed, the kind of drawing-to-your-body motion that looks much like judo pulls (exercise 5), and the lifting and sorting that scapula-strengthening (exercise 7) work can ready you for.

Finally, just because you deserve something nice for doing your own wash, try the total body stretch (exercise 6) to make you feel good, as well as take a little more pressure off your spine.

Prepare your back with exercises 4, 5, 6, 7, and 8.

Being a Student

Remember the myth we discussed earlier, the one that says athletes take chances with their spines and it's much safer to just baby your back? The truth is, fit people have fitter spines, and just sitting around does you no good at all.

It can even do some damage. Spending the whole day hunched at your desk can singlehandedly cause upper-back and neck strain, as Eric, a twenty-four-year-old medical student who obviously hadn't taken back anatomy yet, discovered. He came to me with a pain he described as starting in his neck and going down to his shoulders. It couldn't have been anything he did, Eric assured me, because all he did was sit at his desk day in, day out. In fact, for the last year he had had virtually no time to exercise.

That, of course, was the problem. Eric wasn't able to stretch out his neck muscles, which had consequently grown tighter and tighter. Eventually the cervical muscles supporting his upper spine went into spasm and pinched a nerve, which happened to travel down his back. So did the pain. By simply adding neck stretching (exercise 9) to his daily routine while sitting at the desk, he got rid of his trouble.

If you stay at your desk cradling the phone at your shoulder a good deal, you may well recognize Eric's problem. Your solution will be the same too. You can even do your neck stretches right at your desk. But you *will* have to hang up the telephone first.

Prepare your back with exercise 9.

Ironing

The sweet, humid aroma of clean, steaming clothes may be comforting, and that perfectly pressed collar may be a pleasure to look at, but ironing is still nobody's idea of a good time. Even your back agrees.

So there are two possible solutions. The first is to move nearer a cheap, convenient, and reliable laundry. The other is to continue doing your own ironing, with a back that's prepared for the standing and the constant rowinglike motion.

Rowing? Think about it, your arm going back and forth and back and forth. Row, row, row your iron. Your trunk is rotating, and you're rowing. So you need to start with the Basic 8, of course, and add on the judo pulls (exercise 5), the total body stretch (exercise 6), some scapula strengthening (exercise 7), and the trunk rotations (exercise 8), as well as neck stretches (exercise 9) to unkink the tightness that can come from all of that pushing and pulling.

Prepare your back with exercises 5, 6, 7, 8, and 9.

The Athlete in Us All

As you can see, the athlete's back program for *nonathletes* is really the athlete's back program. Every single way you move your body has a parallel in sport. And though you may reach over your head a little more intensely in a volleyball game than in a supermarket, the muscles used are fundamentally the same and the things that can go wrong with them (and be made right again) are much the same too.

So be creative. Everything you do with your spine can be traced back to some exercise we use to ready athletes for competition. If I've missed an exercise or a motion that concerns you, look at the list of exercises again in chapter 6 and find one that comes close. Then use it to help your back.

Remember, life is motion!

Afterword
Be Smart, Be Active

Congratulations. You've got it!

That's right, you now have all the tools you need to help prevent back pain. And if you're already suffering back pain at the moment, you now know what must be done to get it under control and set yourself on a healthier, more active, pain-free path. Certainly a strong and healthy back is the single most important step any athlete (or *anyone*) can take to try to remain injury-free.

But I can do no more than give you the tools. Now you must put them to work if they are to do you any good.

Remember this old joke?

Q: How many psychiatrists does it take to change a lightbulb?

A: One, but the lightbulb has to really *want* to change.

. . .

I can only lead you to a program that can result in freedom from back trouble. If you really want to do more than wish for a pain-free life, *you* have to do what you now know it takes to change.

You will get out of this book exactly what you put into it. Reading alone achieves nothing, as a patient of mine who had recently joined an aggressive and relatively expensive yoga class was soon reminded. Like most pupils there, he sought better body balance, greater flexibility, and stronger muscles, and the once-a-week classes vigorously worked stiff joints and tendons he'd neglected over years of running.

Most everyone there had bought the instructor's book, which explained the program, and probably an audiotape to inspire at-home workouts. Surely, given all that, they were well on their way to supreme and injury-free suppleness.

Then, at the end of one class halfway through the semester, my patient recounted, one student obviously needed some reassurance. "Excuse me," she said to the instructor. "What will we get out of this program if we come every week but don't practice at home?"

"Nothing," came the blunt reply. "Absolutely nothing."

Honest and correct. And simply reading this book will do nothing for you either. But faithfully put its precepts into action in your life, and watch what happens.

I don't care how busy you are—this is your *back* we're talking about. Make time for the Basic 8 three times a week, minimum. Make time for your specific exercises—the ones that will strengthen you for your particular sports and other activities—three times a week, minimum. If you do, you will have the best possible chance of being pain-free, you'll be in the best position to make the play. If you want to do it, I promise that you can.

Our understanding of the back's structure and the best ways of protecting it can only grow with time, research, and new diagnostic tools. Much exciting work is being done even as you read this book. So if, in the course of your active life, you discover some back preparatory exercise that you find especially helpful that I've not mentioned, please feel free to write me in care of Henry Holt and Company, 115 West 18th Street, New York, New York 10011. I'd love to hear from you.

And most of all, I'd love to hear that your new active lifestyle is back-pain-worry-free.

Enjoy the ride!

Index